Monsieur
Le Vet

Originally published in French in 2015
by Éditions des Arènes under the title
Docteur Fourrure

Monsieur Le Vet

My Life with Animals in Rural France

SYLVAIN BALTEAU

Translated from the French by Barbara Mellor

ICON

Published in the UK in 2016 by
Icon Books Ltd, Omnibus Business Centre,
39–41 North Road, London N7 9DP
email: info@iconbooks.com
www.iconbooks.com

Sold in the UK, Europe and Asia
by Faber & Faber Ltd, Bloomsbury House,
74–77 Great Russell Street,
London WC1B 3DA or their agents

Distributed in the UK, Europe and Asia
by TBS Ltd, TBS Distribution Centre, Colchester Road,
Frating Green, Colchester CO7 7DW

Distributed in the USA by
Publishers Group West,
1700 Fourth Street, Berkeley, CA 94710

Distributed in Canada by
Publishers Group Canada,
76 Stafford Street, Unit 300
Toronto, Ontario M6J 2S1

Distributed in Australia and New Zealand
by Allen & Unwin Pty Ltd,
PO Box 8500, 83 Alexander Street,
Crows Nest, NSW 2065

Distributed in South Africa by
Jonathan Ball, Office B4, The District,
41 Sir Lowry Road, Woodstock 7925

ISBN: 978-178578-057-8

Typeset in Adobe Text Pro by Marie Doherty

Printed and bound in the UK by Clays Ltd, St Ives plc

I dedicate this book to Alice, above all,
to Cécile and to Gaelle.

To my parents and my grandparents.

To all those – teachers,
colleagues, doctors, friends, my brother
and sisters – too numerous to mention,
who have never allowed me to stagnate.

I also dedicate this book to Congélo ('Freezer').

To my beloved old mare Mémé.

And to Oasis.

ABOUT THE AUTHOR

Sylvain Balteau, 36, lives and works in a village in the Haute-Garonne region of France, at the foot of the Pyrenees. He trained as a vet in Toulouse and started keeping a blog of his life in 2007. This is his first book.

Barbara Mellor has over 30 years' experience as a literary translator and editor. Her translation of Agnès Humbert's wartime journal, *Résistance: Memoirs of Occupied France* (Bloomsbury, 2008), was shortlisted for the Scott Moncrieff Prize, and she is also the translator of *A King in Hiding* (Icon, 2015), longlisted for the William Hill Sports Book of the Year Award, 2015.

ACKNOWLEDGEMENT

The publisher and translator would like to thank Rachel Brown BVMS MRCVS of Galedin Veterinary Practice in Kelso in the Scottish Borders for her expert advice on technical matters.

Warning

This book contains graphic accounts of veterinary treatments that some readers may find upsetting.

'I want to be a vet'

Imust have been nine. I was good at school, second in my class. Top of the class was Arnaud, who always managed to scrape in just ahead of me and was forever bragging about it. He was better at this, better at that. He despised the 'magazine for children' that I was brought up on. He read a more sophisticated one, 'that lets readers get behind world news'.

One day our teacher asked us what we wanted to be when we grew up. As always, Arnaud got in first: 'I want to be a vet.'

I'd never even thought about it. Or at least I can't recall now if I had, and I couldn't back then either. I looked at the small dark-haired woman who'd asked the question, the teacher who lit up my last two years at primary school. And quick as a flash I said: 'I want to be a vet.' Arnaud gave me a hard time, obviously. It was *his* idea.

After that I never gave it a second thought. Not until I qualified, fourteen years later.

In the last year at secondary school, I bumped into Arnaud again. He'd moved to another town, far away from us 'country bumpkins'. I was waiting outside school, about to sit a physics exam in which (when they eventually let me leave after sitting it out for an hour) I was to score zero per cent. He was waiting outside a different room, for an exam in history, or geography, or something like that. He went on to business school.

And I became I vet.

Did I become a vet because I love animals?
Being a vet is a vocation, it seems, like being a doctor. According to the dictionary, a vocation is 'a specified occupation, profession, or trade; a special urge, inclination, or predisposition to a particular calling or career'.

But for me it was a calling that started as a feud between two rival nine-year-old teacher's pets.

I'm not convinced that I became a vet 'because I love animals'. Not that I don't love them; for me the question doesn't even arise. But I'm not *in* love with them. This is a misunderstanding that gives rise to some curious conversations with clients.

What do we mean when we talk about loving animals, in any case? They share our lives. They are our witnesses, sometimes our confidants, and they never judge us. They are our companions, at work and play. We put our trust in them, and they have their own personalities, their own qualities and defects of character, whether real or imagined. They are much more than personal belongings, but at the same time – even if sometimes they comfort our loneliness or serve as surrogate family members – they are not people. We may eat them, or we may encourage them to curl up in a ball on our laps. We may bask in the reflected glory of their looks, their intelligence or their breeding.

Do we love them the way we love other people? Or the way we love a good wine? How should we love animals? Many people are besotted with them. Lots of people project their own feelings on to them. Some people used to worship them. So let's say that, yes, I respect and appreciate animals. I love them for what they are. Animals.

I'm not convinced you can be a vet just because you love animals unconditionally. I'm not convinced you can be a vet *if* you love animals unconditionally: as we often hear clients say, 'I could never have been a vet, I love animals too much'. But I *am* convinced that you can't be a vet if you don't love people. Or else you end up as a cynical, embittered alcoholic. So, a vocation? Well, maybe.

In any case, by the time I considered this question seriously it was already too late. I did well enough at school, so I didn't have to have second thoughts about what I wanted to do. I got into vet school at first go, and from then on everything was programmed to go smoothly: if you succeed in getting a place at vet school there's no way they'll let you fail. My vocation consisted, quite simply, of an absence of reflection. Just because you're a straight A student doesn't mean you can't also be a total idiot.

What sort of vet?

So I made it to vet school, but as ever I didn't indulge in any self-reflection. When it came to the first work placements, I turned up all bright-eyed and bushy-tailed. In my first year it was a large equine clinic. I wanted to be a horse vet: I was good at riding and I really liked horses, so naturally I was going to be a horse vet. Then I discovered what a ruthless world it was. Not the horses, but the humans who populate this microcosm of hypocrisy and pettiness. I would never be, could never be, an 'equine' vet; I couldn't ever imagine working in that pretentious and oh-so-exclusive world. Then and there I decided that in future I'd stick to common-or-garden horses and old nags.

So, if I wasn't going to be a horse vet, then I'd be a rural vet. I'd look after cows, do something that mattered. Because it really *does* matter, in the sense that you're treating animals in order to enable other people to earn a living; you're treating them on a case-by-case basis, without any fuss or nonsense, and – most important of all – with humanity. You're working alongside livestock farmers who owe their living to their animals, who live through them and often for them. I wanted to be there for these people who are always there, to go the extra mile with these people who are constantly going the extra mile.

I lasted a year. Just a year of practice before chance, a powerful yearning to get a full night's sleep, and a lack of interest in treating entire herds rather than diagnosing individual animals took me in a different direction. I wanted to look after cows, not herds. I longed for human contact, not Excel spreadsheets.

So it was then that I went into mixed practice. A genuinely mixed practice, working with cows and horses, dogs and cats and any other creatures, great or small, that people might bring in. It had all started off as a childish infatuation. Now I was going to try to go back to fundamentals, to be the kind of vet I'd fantasised about. I wasn't going to be stingy with my time, with either animals or people. And lastly – and this was a long way from being certain – I was going to try to enjoy my work. When I see how many of my colleagues have qualified and then thrown it all in, I see that I'm far from being the only one who questions – frequently – what I'm doing here. I don't blame anyone for leaving the profession: even if you love it, there's stuff that makes you want to run away. I can't imagine what it would be like if you weren't even that interested.

Being a vet

I'm a vet. I'm the archetype of a vet, the sort of vet you see in films and read about in books, the sort of vet who treats every kind of animal.

I look after domestic pets, and I also look after farm animals: cows, pigs, poultry and horses. I may vaccinate a dog, then operate on a bitch with a uterine infection. I may neuter a tomcat, then whisk the cover off the microscope to diagnose a case of the tick-borne disease piroplasmosis. I may X-ray a fracture and then set it, before referring the animal to a specialist vet for surgery. I'm my clients' first resort, and often their last. If they call me out at two o'clock in the morning I'm there every time, no questions asked. To deliver a calf, to do a transfusion on one, to treat a horse with colic.

I work 50 to 60 hours a week. And on top of that I'm on the duty rota, which sometimes means I'm permanently on call.

I employ five people, which I find terrifying. When the accounts are in the red, I wonder how I'm going to pay their wages. And then there are the suppliers. And I'm the one who has to make arrangements when people are off sick, organise maternity cover, and work round locums-who-aren't-as-good-as-the-people-they're-covering-for (but who-are-better-than-nothing-even-so).

I pamper my clients. They all have their expectations, their needs, their personalities and their foibles. I have to know how to listen as they tell me why they've come, then work out the real reason why they're there. They have their preconceptions and their hopes. Their animal may be a badly brought-up toddler. Or a professional tool. Or simply a companion, a pet. It might have come for its first vaccination, it might have come to die. My clients may be intelligent, sensitive, understanding, utterly lost or completely dumb. They may be well off or even wealthy, or they may live in modest circumstances or even on the street. They may be prompt in settling their bills or they may always be late, but they pay my wages. They are often happy with the treatment they receive, and when they aren't, this may be for a very good reason, whether justified or not: when your animal dies you have a right to be angry, even if the vet has done nothing wrong.

People ask me to be a guardian and a witness: my signature and official stamps serve to certify and witness, to all intents and purposes, truly, sincerely and legally. I carry out my duties, whatever the circumstances.

I'm a vet.

I pass on cases to my colleagues, and they pass on cases to me – fortunately. I wouldn't be able to cope on my own. And when I'm at the end of my tether, I seek refuge in the cocoon of my family, or I share my pain online, in the public arena, on my blog.

In this book.

The lottery of life

It was just like any other Monday morning. Rushed, hassled, with the customary bunch of more or less imaginary emergencies that have waited the whole of Sunday because people don't want to call the out-of-hours service, or don't know about it. With the cases admitted over the weekend. With visits, appointments and two operations.

As for me, I was out of the surgery as fast as I could go. It was only a relative emergency, but if I didn't deal with it then and there it would only get worse. When I returned an hour later, I found a scene of chaos: one vet still in the operating theatre and likely to be stuck there for at least another half-hour, another called out to a calving, the waiting room heaving with puppies (whose bright idea was it to book in a litter of puppies for their vaccinations on a Monday morning?), two nurses rushing in all directions, with the constant ringing of the telephone providing a musical accompaniment. I checked the appointments book: Monsieur Gimone had been booked in to have his dog put down an hour earlier.

An hour. An hour that this elderly man had to wait for his dog to die. An hour that he'd been waiting amid all this mayhem for us to put his companion down. I felt quite sick with shame. Quickly I skirted round the waiting room, ignoring the dog breeder and saying hello to another client, and quietly signalled to the old gentleman to come out with me to the car park, where I knew Démon was waiting in the boot of his car.

*

I'd been treating Démon, a Beauceron, for ten years. A year ago, I diagnosed a deadly hemangiosarcoma, a highly invasive form of cancer, in his spleen: it had spread to his liver and was causing bleeding in his abdomen. I'd given him a few days to live. Six months later Monsieur Gimone brought him back, happy to prove me wrong, and I examined a metastatic skin tumour. He was 'getting along fine'. His back was sore and he was too fat – as he had only a few days left I'd told his master to spoil him. But he was 'getting along fine', and as far as Monsieur Gimone was concerned I was a hero, a healer – because I had palpated his dog's abdomen, done a scan and diagnosed cancer, and palpated again; because when I had diagnosed his lumbar pain, I had let my hands linger over the muscles of his back, feeling for spasms and tension.

Afterwards he'd got better. For the hemangiosarcoma I could do nothing. For the arthritic pain it was chiefly my anti-inflammatories that we had to thank. I'd explained this to Monsieur Gimone, but he hadn't listened. When he came to the surgery he would see only me and no one else, because – well, because I was a healer. He had even

warned me to be careful, so as to avoid the evil eye. I'd tried
to set his mind at rest, with a little quip about how arthritis
would be bound to get me in the end.

*

I carried the dog from the car to the examination table.
Monsieur Gimone could barely speak. Démon was leaning
on his side and breathing with difficulty, his abdomen sagging and misshapen. Monsieur Gimone was weeping. He
just said a few last words. Then he asked me to take care of
the body, and he left. Cancer, bleeding, the end.

I inserted the catheter, holding Démon's great head
under my left arm, stroking him and talking to him. On
my own, as the veterinary nurses were still caught up in
a whirl of activity. Démon was stirring a little. I tried to
move away from the table to get the anaesthetic drugs, but
straight away came back without them as I was afraid he
might fall off. I called Julie, one of the nurses, and asked
her to put the phone on silent for a couple of minutes. By
the time I'd fetched the drugs, Démon had managed to
manoeuvre himself into a slightly more upright position.

As Julie held him, she said:

'Monsieur Gimone wanted it to be you, that was why
he waited, he said that if anything needed to be done it had
to be you.'

'*If anything needed to be done?* He told me that he'd
stopped eating, that it was the end.'

Silence. Should I examine him? Yes of course I should
take the time to examine him.

Even in the midst of all that chaos.

So we got Démon up on his paws. He was wobbly, but he managed to stand up. He was panting. But his mucous membranes were pink. His abdomen was sagging, as though distended with liquid. I pierced it with my needle, the one that I'd been going to use to put him to sleep. No blood. I tried again. Still no blood. Fat. I did propriocep-tive tests, to rule out any neurological disorder. Excellent. I pinched his loin muscles hard. He fell over. His blood count was normal. His tumour hadn't bled.

Indecision.

I put the anaesthetic drugs down, picked up the anti-inflammatories: an intravenous injection, since the catheter was in place.

'I'll give him till tonight. Don't tell Monsieur Gimone. If he gets up on his feet, I'll keep an eye on him.'

Julie smiled, and helped me to carry Démon to the small courtyard behind the surgery.

Hours passed, and Démon didn't get up. Worn out by the day, I didn't pay too much attention to him, just giving him a quick glance now and then on my way to the kennels. He wasn't moving, just lying on his front with his proud head held high, alert, panting.

I gave my colleagues a brief rundown: 'I didn't put Démon to sleep, I think he was suffering from severe arthritic pain.'

They signalled their approval without a word, smiling in acknowledgement of the unlikeliness of the story. They run on hope, like I do.

'Hold off on banking Monsieur Gimone's cheque, let's wait till tomorrow!'

*

It was 7.30 that evening, and I was wrapping up the appointments while one nurse did the accounts and another flung the doors open to tackle the cleaning. And then there was a shout:

'Hey, that's your Beauceron! He's got out!'

One of my colleagues was just back from a visit. He was turning the ignition off when he caught sight of the old dog that was now returning our stares from the waste ground behind the surgery. My colleague laughed out loud. It hadn't even occurred to me to tie Démon up. It took me 30 metres to catch up with him; he wouldn't let me get close.

My colleague was creased up: 'Now you'll *have* to call old Gimone!'

He'd be happy, of course he would. But I felt a bit shabby all the same, because I hadn't honoured the agreement I had with my client, because I'd lied to him, because ... because the old boy had been at home crying since that morning. Since the day before, probably.

There was a lump in my throat. I didn't really know what I was going to say. I concocted a few phrases. The ringing tone stopped as someone picked up. A woman's voice, very elderly.

'Madame Gimone?'

'Yes?'

'Hello, this is Sylvain, the vet. I'm calling about ... about something odd that's happened. I'm calling because this morning your husband brought Démon in for me to put him down, and then he left again straight away, and now it turns out that, um ... well, Démon's got better, he's just eaten, and he's run around a bit.'

'Wait, I'll get my husband!'

I'd said it all very quickly, so she wouldn't have a chance to interrupt.

'Roger, it's the vet, he says Démon's been running around, that he's been eating!'

I waited for a moment, feeling a bit emotional, a bit of an idiot, and rather pleased with myself.

'Hello, yes?'

'It's Sylvain. I'm calling because ... this morning, after you left, Julie told me that you wanted me to examine Démon, and I hadn't done that, so I did, and, well, um, it's not his cancer that's the cause of the trouble, it's his arthritis. He was in a lot of pain.'

'Démon's in pain?'

'Not now, not much, I've given him some injections, and now he's better – I mean I haven't cured his cancer, but he's feeling better, he's managed to eat, and he even tried to run away.'

'To run away? Démon?'

Incredulity.

'Errrm ... yes, we'd forgotten to shut the doors, but I caught him. I had to run after him.'

'He had to run after him!' He was shouting now.

Then he spoke into the receiver again:

'And he's eaten?'

'Yes, he's had a bowl of food, and a drink, and a pee, and, well, there you are, I'm very sorry, I didn't want to call you earlier as I didn't want to raise your hopes, just in case it didn't work out.'

'And he can come home?'

'Yes, with some pills, yes. Because, well, he's still got cancer, but it's like it was before: since the bleeding stopped a year ago he could go on for another day, or another week, or another six months.'

*

Monsieur Gimone came back to collect his dog.

He thanked me, in tears, grumbling as always about the cost of the medication, saying that living was no cheaper than dying.

Then he shook my hand, holding it in his for a long time.

*

If it hadn't been for the nurse, Démon would have been put to sleep.

Pirate

A woman of about 30 comes into the surgery. She looks confused and a little embarrassed.

She's elegantly dressed in a short skirt and blouse, her long hair is immaculately styled, and she's carrying a shoebox.

'Excuse me, I have an appointment for, um ...'

'Yes, for the rat? No problem, follow me.'

I take the lid off the box and pick up the creature. A fine large variegated male, a nice old boy. I hold him under his shoulders, my thumb and first finger around his thorax, his back paws dangling. His long tail gyrates while his nose quivers on a level with mine. He makes vague efforts to get away by pushing with his front paws. One of his eyes is punctured. Blood has seeped under the socket and coagulated. He's cleaned some of it away.

'Um, I ... It's not my rat. It belongs to my neighbour's son. He came round to my house just now with the creature in his hands. He's eight. His father had told him that if he wanted to make it better he should take it to the woods and let it go.'

*

The bastard.

He's not the first. One day a little girl of six came running in with her hamster, all on her own. The hamster was dying. I was obliged to have a consultation with a six-year-old child, explain to her that her hamster was certainly going to die, try all the same to save it because I couldn't just let it die, talk to her about death. Tell her that we would give it an injection to stop the pain, and then let it slip away. Dither between hollow and inaccurate clichés – 'It'll go to sleep' – and the blunt truth for which I would have to accept the consequences. Was it my job to explain to a six-year-old child that no, the vet couldn't save her hamster, that he couldn't even suggest anything except killing it? To explain to her about death?

Anyway, so I made her a sweet little coffin for her hamster, from a small cardboard box for antibiotics.

To make matters worse she insisted on paying, holding out her pocket money, a heap of small change. I told her that in this surgery it was grown-ups who paid. I wasn't going to let her father off the hook.

*

As I listen to this woman, I'm shaking with anger. She notices, says she's sorry. I tell her I'm sorry, quickly tell her the story of the little girl and the hamster.

'You know I'm happy to pay, I mean it's not my rat, he's not even my son, but please don't send the bill to his father ...'

*

So I decide to do everything I can, which shouldn't cost too much. A rat shouldn't suffer too badly from losing an eye. Anyway, it seems blithely unconcerned, wriggling about and running up and down my arm, not exactly what you'd call disabled. She'll come back for it tonight.

We keep it, clean it up, put it in a gauze-lined cage to sleep, take time to give it a proper clean-up – and I'm not convinced that any of this is justified. Antibiotics. A dressing, a bandage over its eye and round its head. It looks like a pirate.

As for the bill, she can pay as much or as little as she wants. Whatever. The rat will be just fine, anyway.

Midnight

The cow is jammed between a barrier and the wall of an old building off the cowshed where there's a stone feeding trough and a gnarled wooden manger. A thick carpet of fresh straw, light from two big yellow bulbs. It's warm, hot almost. Somewhere in one of the hay bales a kitten mews. The blonde cow has been straining for hours, but to no avail, a fine large cow that has seen other births and that shouldn't need any help. What will I find this time? There's no let-up between calvings, all of them different, constant, relentless and exhausting. There won't be any rest for a few weeks yet, not until the season's over.

I'm inside the softness of a cow's birth canal again, silent, too tired to talk. I might have made a bit of small talk on auto-pilot, but my head's somewhere else, at the end of my arm, at the tips of my fingers as they explore the vagina and then the cervix, while the cow starts to strain again. I'm not really concentrating, just confident and relaxed. I enjoy calving on this farm. And in any case, with a pelvis like this it hardly matters what's inside, it will emerge in the natural way. I'd put money on a uterine torsion, a twisting of the uterus that's not uncommon in cows.

I push my arm in deeper and turn my hand anti-clockwise until it's resting on the calf's head, still enveloped in the placental membranes. It's alive, I've got a good hold, this should be quick. The uterus, with its hundreds of litres of calf, mucus and damp membranes, suspended by two ligaments that are too lax, has spun on itself. The twisted uterus is constricting the birth passage and preventing the calf from passing through it, but by a stroke of luck the cervix seems to be dilated.

The mother pants and pushes, twists her body and stamps her hooves; the farmer holds her tail while I lay my hand quite flat on the calf's neck. Its mother must weigh 700 kilos. Luckily I'm tall.

It's a knack you learn that becomes habitual, a powerful, continuous movement that culminates in a final push, using the combined strength of your arm and your back. Sometimes for a moment, as now, sometimes for ten minutes or so. With one last rocking movement the calf is facing down the birth canal, feet down and head between its front legs; I rupture the sac and allow the fluids to flow with the contractions. The cervix is well dilated, the canal is very wide, I'm guessing the calf's a female, a good size but not too big. She'll pass through.

My hands are on her cannon bones and I can feel her trembling, tiny spasms as though she were shaking her head. No time to lose. Gently, powerfully, I pull the little hooves towards the vulva, damp yellow and ivory against the slippery coat, with a sickly sweet smell. A little blood and a lot of amniotic fluid on my overalls and all down my arms. It's fine, it's warm, I feel good, so good, here, holding this newborn in position while the farmer runs to fetch the calving ropes that I wrap around her legs. It's a good hold. He positions the calving jack, while I very slowly pass the neck of the uterus over the newborn's head. The hooves have now emerged, and I suspend myself from the ropes, my body completely straight, my feet wedged in the straw between the cow's hind legs. I imagine I'm holding the strings of a kite, effortlessly, my head 70 centimetres from the ground and nearly horizontal, pulling downwards and backwards, in time with the mother's contractions.

Above me, barely a metre away from my eyes, I can see the lips of the vulva spreading to reveal the tip of a tongue, then a wet nose and a muzzle covered in mucus, eyes, a forehead, ears ... The farmer hurries to position the jack, but there's no need, the calf is being drawn out by the traction of my weight, as I bend my legs a little to stop myself from falling over.

Out come the shoulders, then the thorax. The farmer has left the jack in the straw and is getting ready to hold the calf's hind legs, while I kneel to receive the newborn. She breathes in, exhales a damp and mucous breath, and shakes her head as we hang her upside down to expel the last of the mucus. Her mother moans and lows, calls her and looks over her shoulder at these two bipeds tending to her calf.

One last descent into the birth canal, empty now: a little blood, a cervix in perfect condition, a soft vagina with no tears, no damage to arteries. After a last look once we've cleaned up, I can go home to bed. The calf is already trying to stand up, her mother dribbles and froths as she licks her in a trance, watching us out of the corner of her eye while the farm dogs curl up on their straw bed behind the wall. An owl hoots. In the feeding trough the kitten mews again. The calves are nearly all asleep; two of them follow me with their great cow eyes. Time for bed.

Barter

It's half past nine in the evening. I'm on call tonight and all over the weekend, and I'm flicking between the internet and a book that doesn't look too promising. Basically I'm bored stiff, but not so bored that I'm actually hoping for a call. Which is going to happen anyway. I stare for ten seconds as the telephone rings and flashes, signalling that a call is being transferred.

'Out-of-hours service, hello?'

'Er ... is that the vet?'

'Yes it is ...'

'It's my piglet, I've got a piglet, he's a week old and I've had him for five days, I've just got home from work and he's lying on the floor and there's a cigarette crushed on the floor and he's not good and I've given him mouth-to-mouth can you imagine I gave my piglet mouth-to-mouth and I massaged his heart and then he came round but he's not at all good what shall I do I massaged him and there's a cigarette all mashed up beside him and what shall I do can you come and see him?'

'Ermmm ...'

'I've been feeding him with pig milk powder from the agricultural cooperative and in the beginning his mother fed him the bloke told me that he should have immunity but now I think he's chewed up that cigarette and I've brought him round twice I've just put him in front of a little space heater to warm him up he's frozen.'

'OK, well if it's as bad as that I'll just have to come ...'

*

I'm floundering, stumped, totally at sea. In fact the conversation went on much longer than that. All I managed to get in were a few 'ums' and 'ers', and the occasional 'It's not the cigarette.'

I can't work it out, but the guy is genuinely distraught. He doesn't sound as though he has learning difficulties, but from the way he talks about his piglet I can tell he's not used to dealing with pigs. And this piglet seems to enjoy a peculiar position, half farm animal, half pet. If this were a sick and motherless week-old piglet destined for the sausage factory, a farmer wouldn't bother to do anything. The cost of a night call-out would be enough to buy five piglets, if not more.

But if it's a pet ... I just can't make it out. And he seems to want me to make a visit, without actually asking me to.

I'm uncertain, I don't want to upset him, he's made an emergency call, I'll go. But will he be able to pay for the call-out?

'OK, well then, if it's as bad as that, I'm on my way.'

'But how much will it cost?'

Bingo. I feel a bit embarrassed, but he's broached the subject, so much the better.

'About 50 euros ... but ...'

Silence.

'50 euros? But I haven't got 50 euros!'

He's not saying, 'but that's daylight robbery' or 'but that's too much'. No, he's saying, 'but I haven't got 50 euros'.

'Leave it, I'm on my way, we'll sort it out. I'll be there in ten minutes at the outside.'

He lives not far from my house. What would I have done if he'd been 40 kilometres away?

He lives on an old farm that's he's in the middle of doing up. He apologises for the mess. He takes me up to the first floor, into a small bathroom where a space heater is blowing hot air. Lying under a blanket, in the full blast of the hot air, is a pink piglet with black markings. It's so sweet. On the way up, the guy tells me that a friend gave it to him because its mother had crushed the rest of the litter.

The piglet is dying. Its breathing is laboured, its heartbeat is far too slow, and it's so hypothermic that its temperature doesn't even register on the thermometer. Its skin is lightly mottled with violet. I don't know what's wrong with it, I just know that it's going to die. That it would probably already be dead if the bearded bloke kneeling beside me hadn't made such desperate efforts to bring it back to life. I tell him. He punches the ground with his fist, wants to know why. I'd struggle to find an explanation for him.

He appears to have done everything right, but the piglet

won't survive. I suggest we should help it on its way, inject it with a large dose of anaesthetic. To make it quicker.

He comes out to the car with me, and we talk in the darkness of the farmyard, lit by the courtesy light in the back of the car, while I fill the syringe. I'd known this was why I was here.

As I get ready to inject the anaesthetic, he stops me.

'It's my piglet. I want to.'

He sounds firm, determined. And sad.

Very simply, I show him how to do an intramuscular injection.

He doesn't hesitate for a second.

The little piglet's emerald-green eyes roll back in its cartoon-like snout.

*

'What do I owe you, doctor?'

Look, my friend, you don't owe me a thing. I came to put your piglet down because I'm experienced enough – or cynical enough – to know that there was nothing else I could do. To make sure it didn't suffer, to make sure I wouldn't have to leave you on your own with a dying newborn.

I don't say this, but I dodge the question, tell him to leave it.

He won't have it, of course. So we carry on chatting under the stars, about the sheep that he's just been to collect, the pigs that he'd like to breed, that sort of thing. And then I set off home, taking with me two slices of inedible cake (sorry) and an old stool. Because there was no way I could say no.

He was shaking.

Sunday

It's Sunday. I'm on call, trailing my mobile with me wherever I go, even to the toilet, but I'm at home. I've been on call for two days non-stop. My last afternoon off was Thursday, my next one will be Tuesday. The days have been busy, the nights not so bad.

It's half past seven in the morning and I'm in bed. The phone rings. Top volume, action stations. A woman's voice. Young.

'Out-of-hours service, hello?'

'Oh doctor it's awful, my guinea pig's got a tick, I'm so frightened!'

What?!

'Right. Ermm, that's not really serious. You'll just have to remove it.'

'But how??? There are the children!'

'Ah. Yes. Well then ... Hold on a minute, I'll take your number. I'll call you back when I'm at the surgery.'

I stagger off to get a pen and paper, write down her number.

'*Merci docteur!*'

Half past seven and now I'm wide awake. I could have told her where to get off. I didn't even think of it. On weekday mornings people never wake me up with such dumb questions. Only on Sundays and holidays. Later on, when I go to the clinic to check on my surgery cases, I'll get her in with her guinea pig and its tick. Show her how to remove it, sell her a tick remover, not even charge her the out-of-hours rate. Still, what a halfwit.

I let my dogs out, have breakfast, down a coffee, log on to Twitter. I'll go to the surgery early, I've got some serious cases in the kennels, not that they're urgent, but here on my own I'm going round in circles, getting stressed out. I read a bit – my beloved *Veterinary Internal Medicine* by Stephen Ettinger – take none of it in, pick up my keys, pull the door to behind me.

I'm off to vote now, quickly, as I can't be sure I'll have the time later on. At the polling station there's a handful of elderly villagers and a plate of crêpes. I give a few quick handshakes, wolf down the crêpe offered to me by the lady mayor, and shoot off again, waving my mobile as my alibi.

Emergencies, that sort of thing.

*

It's nine o'clock when I arrive at the clinic. The dog that should have died three days ago is doing well. Really well. The phone rings, a labrador that's off his food, down in the dumps, not himself. It could be a case of piroplasmosis, caught from a tick bite. I won't make his master wait. You can't take any risks with piroplasmosis. It's endemic in this region, it's the season, it's a killer. While I wait for him to arrive I call the guinea pig woman and tend to my major surgery patient. The cat that had surgery last night is just fine, there are no concerns, he's purring away peacefully in his cage with his cushion, his bowl, his litter and his morphine medication. Unlike many cats, he hasn't even disturbed his catheter. I leave him in peace. He's a soothing presence.

*

The labrador and his owner arrive before long, so there's no time to take out the dog that's had surgery. The young lab, usually irrepressible, barely wags his tail. His master was right to bring him in. There's no fever, the clinical examination is normal, the piroplasmosis smear negative, the dog's not even really ill. But there's something.

He's clearly in pain. The stomach is soft, but when I palpate it he gives me an accusing look.

'Does he scoff any old rubbish, this young rascal?'

'Um, no, he stopped all that a few months ago.'

I pull on a glove, making it snap like they do on the telly. A finger in the rectum, I can feel hard bits and there are drops of blood. Dumb dog. What's he gone and eaten? I scowl at the poo: streaks of blood.

Analgesics, antibiotics as a precaution, paraffin; if he's not better tomorrow I'll see him again: I don't think I'll need to operate on this chap.

Meanwhile, as I'm dealing with the labrador, the guinea pig woman has arrived. I remove the tick with the little

hooked instrument that works so brilliantly, show her how
to do it. Four euros fifty for waking me up on a Sunday,
for being reassured even if there was absolutely nothing to
worry about. It seems crazy to me, but I can't see any other
way round it. I send the woman and her guinea pig home.
What can you say? I save lives. I tell myself that I understand why some doctors don't offer an out-of-hours service
any more, since the genuine emergencies go straight to
Accident and Emergency anyway, which just leaves them
with dumb stuff. Like this.

*

It's eleven o'clock, and my neighbour arrives with his
dog. We arranged the appointment yesterday. The dog,
an elderly setter, had helped himself to a bowlful of fat
the day before, and it was having trouble working its way
through his system. I wanted to check on him, even if yesterday everything seemed to be happening normally. The
old dog has already had hepatitis, pancreatitis, prostati-
tis and uveitis (an eye inflammation), so all we need is a
merry cocktail of all that topped off by raging indigestion.
Dog-itis. No poo since yesterday, but no vomiting either. I
do an X-ray to check there's no blockage. Nothing to report
apart from his arthritis and the lead shot he got peppered
with years ago. I give him some analgesics; we'll see how
he is tomorrow.

I take my in-patient – a griffon – out for his walk, and
inform a chap who's found a dog that its owner has had the
sense to have it microchipped. A beep, the chip is read,

I send him back home straight away. This too is a public service: I never charge for this sort of thing, except when I have to keep the dog for a while until its owner can come and fetch it.

Finally it's midday, and I've done with my emergencies. I check my drips, do a tour of the surgery, lock the door.

Outside the little town hall, also a polling station, a crowd of people has gathered in the sunshine. There's a queue stretching between the baker's, the tobacconist and the town hall. But here there are no crêpes.

*

Ten to two, and for once I've managed to have lunch. The phone rings again.

A calving. This client couldn't be more different from the guinea pig woman. I grab a lollipop in place of dessert. Watermelon flavour, my favourite.

A twenty-minute drive, stopping off at the surgery to pick up the embryotome, just in case.

On the way the phone rings again. A dog with a torn claw. Painful, obviously, but not serious. I give the woman some advice on what to do, but she still wants me to see it. I explain to her that I'm on my way to a major emergency, that I might be a couple of hours. That I'll call her back.

Draughts whistle through the little cowshed. It's freezing cold despite the sunshine, but I've got my calving gear to shield me from the wind. The client doesn't often see me dressed up like this. With his fifteen Salers cattle we never have to do any obstetrics. Salers practically always give birth unattended. But he's done the right thing: he's spotted a cow that's looks sick, moved her to a sheltered spot, pushed the calf that was already half engaged in the birth canal back inside her.

I pull on my gloves, plunge my arms into the warmth of the birth canal. The young cow doesn't like it, but she doesn't protest. There's the calf, anterior presentation, normal. One foreleg was bent backwards, the farmer says. A minor thing, but still, when you're not used to it ... What concerns me is the emptiness, the feeling of space in the uterus. Normally the uterus hugs the calf closely, even if it's slack through exhaustion, and there are no expanses of space. But here my hands seem to be feeling their way through a cathedral of mucous membranes. And I can make out the left kidney too clearly, and the belly, there at the bottom. Ruptured. I take my gloves off to get to the bottom of it, to feel the detail: it's catastrophic. The cow is torn, from the vagina to halfway down the uterus probably, with the cervix hanging loose in the middle. By a stroke of good fortune the arteries are intact and the calf is still alive. I slide my fingers over the ends of the tear, I can feel an ovary in passing.

Oh well.

I pull a gloomy face. On seeing my expression, the farmer and his wife look glum too.

'OK. Your calf has tried to come out via a C-section, all by itself. It's managed to open up the uterus, though the incision is pretty much the work of a beginner, but the peritoneum, muscles and hide are a complete bloody shambles. I'll finish the job off: I'll open up here [indicating her flank], we'll get the calf out through the hole it's made, and I'll close everything up again. It's a hell of a mess, it'll take a couple of hours or more, it might not work, she could die of shock, or she could get peritonitis in the next few days. The calf should be OK. I'll need two buckets of water, cold will do.'

They hesitate. They're shocked – they've never seen anything like this – as well as reassured by my pathetic excuses for jokes. I know what I have to do, I feel confident, and they can sense it. They trust me.

At times like this you feel a strange sensation of power. Every country vet has had a go at this sort of surgery. With varying degrees of success, I can only imagine. It's not taught at vet school. It can't be taught, full stop. It's a total shambles, you never know what you're going to find when you open the animal up, you have your little surgical kit and your hands, and you're completely on your own. It's exhilarating. Especially when you've done it before and you know it can work.

The first time it happened to me, I had to make it up as I went along. Since then I've refined my style a little. This morning I removed a tick from a guinea pig. Now the life of a calf and a cow depend on what I'm about to do. Even if I do well, she could die. But I have to try. You always have to try.

While I scrub the cow, anaesthetise her flank, tie her back legs and insert a nose clamp, Madame returns with the buckets of water. I set out my surgical kit, get out my suture material and my scalpel, disinfect my hands and arms, explain to Monsieur how to pull the calf and when I will present it to him. He's nervous, and rolls a cigarette that he'll light a hundred times during the operation.

I make the incision, dodge a kick that's fairly feeble and in any case hampered by the stirrups. A Salers hide is thick. It's the first time I've operated on one, I think. Beneath the hide, two fine layers of muscle, then the peritoneal cavity. I push the stomach towards the front, slip my arm behind it. There's the opening. From the middle of the left uterine horn to the vagina. More or less straight. The calf is reasonably well positioned for an extraction. I pull out its legs, hold them out to the farmer, who positions the nooses, and with my help pulls the calf out without any difficulty. The animal is shaken, has difficulty breathing. A shot of analeptics to stimulate the nervous system helps. I observe it for three minutes before going to wash and disinfect my hands again. Now things are about to get serious.

We're on a small country lane, and the cowshed is open to the road. With the election going on, there's a terrific amount of coming and going. Just like outside the town hall, people stop to have a chat. Old people, young people, a little six-year-old girl who wants to know if it hurts the cow, and why the calf is trembling like that. She's cold too. A woman gets a blanket out of the boot of her car to put over the calf, and helps the little girl put her jacket on.

I'm wearing my dustbin-green overalls, with my arms plunged up to the elbows in the abdomen of a cow. There's no way I can bring the uterus out, even partially, so I'm doing the stitches completely blind. I call it finger-suturing, as I prick my fingers every time to stop the point of the needle. I tighten my continuous suture over my fingers, cut into my joints. As I write this, I can count a dozen cuts and puncture wounds on my fingers. The only painful ones are on the second joints of each index finger, over which the thread passes when I tighten it. The first continuous suture is the riskiest. The wide ligament and the placental debris make it awkward. Damn fool calf. It takes me nearly three-quarters of an hour to finish this first suture. Not completely watertight, but close. The second, buried deep, takes me close on half an hour. Oh what fun it is to do a continuous suture between the serous membrane and the muscle membrane without stitching through the mucous membrane, when you've got both arms inside the cow and can see precisely nothing. Tell me about it.

An old woman watches me as I work, smiling. She used to have cattle, a while back, before my time. Not a single person talks about politics, not one. They chat about the neighbour's little daughter, about the sheep, about the rain, about how fine the weather is, about a christening, about how the grass is growing, about the calf and how he's quite big, but not that big. They talk about everything, about all the most important things in their lives. They talk about the vet who was here before me, who's dead now. The Pyrenees are magnificent in the sunshine.

I feel useful, even if – when it comes down to it – they're not that interested in me.

I've finished my continuous sutures. A man, the

farmer's father I think, wants to know how much thread I needed. Two and a half metres. He can't believe it. Someone who I didn't see arriving or leaving comes back with a bottle of colostrum borrowed from the dairy farmer next door. It's come out of the freezer and has been warmed up over a pan of hot water.

I empty a bottle of penicillin into the mother's abdomen. More out of habit than conviction, but it's an eloquent gesture. Just as good as an intramuscular injection. First muscular continuous suture, second muscular continuous suture. This time it goes very quickly. I suture the hide, a neat job in satin stitch, all the while dodging kicks from the patient, who doesn't appreciate my artistry – the anaesthetic's effect on the skin is always wearing off by the end.

I'm done.

All that remains is to clean up, and wash off the dried blood. I'm plastered with it. The water in the buckets is hot. I don't feel the cold particularly, but I could weep for joy.

*

Everyone's gone. But the calf still has its blanket.

I explain a bit about post-operative care to the farmer and his wife. Nothing very complicated. Their confidence is tragic.

It's a lovely day, even in the teeth of the wind.

In the car, the mobile reels off its messages. An injured cat. I'm thinking about the woman whose dog has torn its claw out when I get a call from a hunter: one of his dogs has just had its stomach ripped open by a wild boar. I make appointments for both dog and cat at the same time. The first to arrive will be the first on the operating table, while the second will be hospitalised. I call back about the dog with its injured paw, apologise, and explain to its owner that there are other animals that I have to treat first. She accepts this without a fuss, and asks for a few words of advice. Tomorrow she'll go to her own vet (who doesn't offer an out-of-hours service).

At the surgery I wait a little, tidy up a few papers, squint at my paperwork from afar. The tax return. I log on to Twitter. The usual babble. It's spring.

The hunter arrives first. A good big hunting dog, like a Bleu de Gascogne basset hound with a lot of other things thrown in, with a fine wound on its upper leg. And a small hole in the abdomen. Easily enough to justify a general anaesthetic. I've inserted the catheter and attached the drip by the time the cat arrives. A hefty tomcat, clearly half-feral if not more, with a nasty wound on its neck, probably an old abscess that's ruptured. Pretty disgusting. I talk to the woman for a few minutes, suggest I should take advantage of the anaesthetic to neuter him. She agrees – that'll teach him to get into fights, she says – so I'll keep him in overnight and she can pick him up tomorrow.

It's past five o'clock, and I still have two operations to do.

*

The big dog is quickly anaesthetised. The wound on his leg barely needs stitching, but a drain won't hurt. The hole in his abdomen turns out to be nothing to worry about. Half an hour later I leave the dog to come round and give his owner advice and explanations about the aftercare he'll need.

It's six o'clock when I attempt to anaesthetise the cat. I manage to do the injection, but – as a tough and semi-wild tom – he tries to rip me to shreds, wriggles out of my grasp and destroys the prep room before finding a safe spot under a cupboard. We've deliberately left enough space there to make a cat hideaway, precisely for cases like this. While I wait for the anaesthetic to take effect I pass the time in tending to my big hunting dog and chatting away online.

Catheter in, drip attached. The phone rings again. A very sick calf. I tell the farmer I'll call in after I've finished operating. Dealing with the abscess takes a good twenty minutes, the neutering five more. I put the cat in a cage, check everything's OK, and I'm off.

*

The calf is a ten-minute drive away. It's twenty past seven by the time I examine it. Severe pain, bad enough to finish it off. Nasty haemorrhagic diarrhoea, high fever. Colic, salmonella or coccidiosis? I'm inclined to the latter, but bits of fibrin and necrosis in the diarrhoea make me less certain. It's very sick, in any case. Unsure, I treat for both bacteria and protozoa, take a specimen, and above all ease the pain. At a quarter to eight I'm back at the surgery, decanting the diarrhoea for a coproscopy. At eight o'clock I have the result. Massive coccidiosis.

I don't call the farmer. He'll come tomorrow anyway for the rest of the treatment – if the calf survives the night, which is far from certain.

I walk the hospitalised dog, a great soppy Alaskan malamute. We have a new President of the Republic, Twitter babbles on at such a rate that I've lost track, and the cat I operated on yesterday is still here. Full of beans. The one whose abscess I sorted and whose cojones I've just cut off is coming round gently.

I leave a message for the malamute's owners, and the prep room for the cleaner. In a woeful state. I feel for her, but I just can't do any more.

I lock the door. In the distance, cars hoot in celebration.

*

When I get home it's twenty to nine. Time for an early night. Tomorrow's a busy day.

Entente cordiale

He's in the waiting area. He looks tired and sad, with his dog, a Pyrenean shepherd, on the knees. He's lost in his thoughts, and as he moves his lips silently his magnificent moustache quivers in sympathy. He's British, a retired RAF officer.

I see a lot of British people and their pets in my everyday practice. Families who have moved here for ... a different life?

Often they've bought a dilapidated old house and refurbished it. People in the area would complain because this pushed prices up much higher than they used to be. But the people who sold to them weren't complaining, I imagine, nor the people they employed to do the work. And let's be honest. We love to see these old ruins brought back to life, as beautiful farms with lovely gardens and magnificent stone walls.

Some of them are retired. The younger ones are ex-members of the military, the older ones used to be teachers, secretaries or lawyers, or they had a shop or worked in a factory in some London suburb. I see artists, too, a sculptor, and even a crazy musician. Listening to their accents, I often wonder where they come from.

Some of them are rich. That's what we often used to think: 'Rich enough to buy stone houses and to rebuild them.' Well, now I know better. Those of modest means have had a hard time as the falling rate of exchange has dramatically shrunk their pensions. Some have even packed up and left, or have stayed on a part-time basis, or have sent their partner back to the UK to earn an income.

And they have pets. Not all of them, I suppose. It's possible that I have an over-representation of pet owners among my clients, is it not?

In our practice, all the vets and half the nurses speak fluent or nearly fluent English. So British pet-owners sometimes drive a long way to see us.

When I hear an English accent in the waiting room, I always start speaking English. I try not to, and it would be better to ask first. Some of my British clients speak very fluent French, but I can't help myself. I start off in English, then when they answer in French I stop to think. We often finish up like this: I speak English, they answer in French; that way we can both be sure of what the other is going to understand.

Dogs and cats don't care anyway.

She was what, 86? She always came in her old Fiat Punto, her husband driving, half-blind, totally deaf. Always enthusiastic when he shook my hand. He was 95. She was a famous dachshund breeder, and she always complained when she didn't get her tea or her whisky on time. She was like something out of Monty Python. I miss her a lot.

When I'm tired, at the end of the day, I start speaking English to the wrong people. To the nurse. To my computer. On a prescription. To a very old French man with an unusual intonation because of his deafness (but he didn't hear me, so he didn't take offence).

They were quite young. They had a business in the UK, they lived here for eight years but in the end they left France, with their five children. They left their friends, and the beautiful watermill they'd totally rebuilt, because the tax on foreign incomes had gone up so high they couldn't afford it. I miss them. I miss the way they used to come on the green motorbike they loved to ride through the hills and along the rivers. I still remember the day I went to the mill to put down their labrador, the old lady they cherished so much.

Speaking English is often a bit of a game: finding the right word (or the right way to pronounce it when eyebrows knit in puzzlement), asking people, checking Google translate.

He drives trucks for British rock stars. He doesn't earn much, and spends most of it on his animals. He's always six months late paying his bills, he's always six months late with everything. He comes to us from quite a long way off, because, he tells me (making me blush in the process), we care.

So I take care, every day, of British cats and dogs, or of French cats and dogs belonging to British people. Though 'Englishness' is something I shouldn't assume too fast, I guess.

That day was a tough one. There they were, a gay couple with a tabby alley cat, and there I was, giving them a laborious explanation of my diagnosis. Either the cat had nothing but a minor virus, or else he had a condition that was fatal. Quite a difference, and I was trying to make an educated guess, wondering whether it was worth while doing more costly examinations. I gave them a very long talk in English; they listened without even a nod or a frown. Since they didn't say anything, I finally began to wonder. Maybe I was wrong? Maybe I'd got the wrong accent? Maybe they were German, or some other nationality?

So I asked them:

'You're English, aren't you?'

They answered, slowly, coolly, with a grin.

'We're Scots.'

They were Scots, and they had a peculiar sense of humour. When they left, I didn't know if they were grateful for the consultation and explanations, or if they were simply laughing at me.

So now I don't assume that people are English, and if I'm in doubt I ask if they are English-speaking. And every day I see English-speaking, or rather English-understanding, dogs and cats.

For the rituals of the Pet Travel Scheme, the visit we have to do for every dog, cat or ferret that's about to cross the Channel.

For vaccinations.

For small wounds, or big ones.

For serious diseases, or simple colds.

I groom.

I pet.

I diagnose.

I care, the best I can.

A good death

Madame Devèze was 59 at the time. I'd always find her surrounded by her cows, pitchfork in hand. That day she looked imposing in the rays of the rising sun, with frost glittering on the straw in the animal stalls and the breath of her blonde cows rising in billowing clouds in the half-light of the cowshed.

I loved her big calloused hands and the way she had of buttonholing me whenever she had an argument with her son, a great strapping lad more interested in sowing, ploughing and making silage than in feeding and handling the cows.

Here, she was the farmer. The others – her husband with his pastis, her son with his tractor – were mere farmhands.

'The men frighten the cows!' she would explain.

She was the one who'd call me out for emergencies, who'd send her son to the surgery to collect the medication, who'd write the names of the drugs and products on a bit of card or a feed label, which he would clutch in his great paws and read with a look of amazement.

She'd always tell me that she wasn't going to carry on until she was 65, that she only had another year to go, and that she'd make voluntary contributions for the rest of her pension, or not, in fact she didn't really know, as she didn't really know what she was entitled to. Like many other women in her position, she'd grown up on a farm and had taken over the work of the farm herself well before anyone took any interest in wives like her, wives who ran farms that were declared in their husband's names. Who knew how they toiled away, who took into account their countless hours of work, their 80-hour weeks with no prospect of holidays, no trips away, no time off? Nowadays most elderly couples who want to be able keep their cows put the farm in the name of the wife, who hasn't paid any contributions and so doesn't have a pension.

And she'd be there, with her pitchfork, fretting over a lame cow or agonising about a calf that needed a transfusion.

'So, Balteau, how are you today?'

Madame Devèze didn't speak with the local accent; she had an unusual and unmistakable voice, and a curious way of speaking, as though she always suspected that people might be laughing at her, or trying to take her for a ride. A life spent staking out her patch.

'Very well, Madame. And you?'

A handshake, a direct smile, no hidden agenda. Sunrise. A herd of cows. Good reasons to be up at dawn, or earlier.

'Oh, well, OK, but I get a bit tired, the work's never

done, you know how it is', she replied, gesturing with her pitchfork.

'So I see. Couldn't your son do that with his tractor?'

'Not in among the cows!'

Of course not.

'But I've got to the point where I've had enough, you know, and on top of that I get this wretched pain, tight across my chest and shooting up my left arm, it's so annoying!'

She accompanied this description with a gesture that was both expansive and eloquent.

I blanched.

'A pain that starts in your heart and travels up your arm? A feeling like you're being crushed, or suffocated?'

'Oh, yes, just like that.'

Her smile was disarming.

'But – surely you must be joking. No?'

'Why? It's nothing serious, is it?'

Really?

'The pain you're describing is typical of the early signs of a heart attack, and here you are with your pitchfork, turning the hay all alone, in among the cows? You must leave all this and see a doctor straight away!'

'Oh, well. That's all I need! Never mind that, come and see this cow, she can't seem to deliver her calf ...'

I pulled on my gloves, protesting all the while.

'And then you'll go to the doctor, won't you? As soon as I've seen to the cow?'

'But it would be a good death, wouldn't it? In the hay, in among the cows?'

'It would be a completely idiotic death more like, at 59, in among all the muck and manure. And what *is* a good death, anyway?'

'Oh well, I expect you're right ...'

She'd dropped the familiar *tu* now, and was using the more formal *vous*.

'But there's no need to worry, Balteau, I take my husband's pills, I took some this morning, they gave me hot flushes but I'm all right now.'

'You took ... What exactly have you taken?'

'Oh, trin something, tritin ...?'

'Trinitrine! Without a prescription? But you must be completely mad! You'll be keeling over in the muck with your cows if you carry on with this nonsense! You shouldn't mess around with drugs like that. They might be completely the wrong thing for you, I don't know. And on top of that you've just told me you've had the symptoms of a heart attack!'

*

In point of fact, I don't know much more about heart attacks than you can pick up from watching medical dramas on television. Animals don't have heart attacks.

I spent another ten minutes arguing with her before I left. I was worried. After lunch I was on the verge of calling her doctor. Then I was called out on a few visits and it went clean out of my mind.

The next day I came into the waiting room to find one of the secretaries and a woman I didn't know deep in conversation.

'Imagine, she told the reception desk at the hospital ...'

I barged in without a second thought.

'What is it? Who's in hospital?'

'Oh doctor, did you not hear what happened to my sister?'

'Her sister is Madame Devèze', the secretary intervened.

'Is she OK?'

'She's absolutely fine, she's getting some rest, she went to the hospital because you gave her such a fright!'

'No bad thing either.'

'They're keeping her in for a little while, she's had all sorts of tests and they've started her on some drugs already ...'

'Have they now.'

'But you'll never guess what she told them at the hospital! When they asked her the name of the doctor who'd referred her, she told them it was you. Since they didn't know you, they asked if you were a locum, and she said no, that you'd told her she should go and tell them that she'd been taking her husband's pills. That you were her vet!'

The old cat

The elderly man sits in the waiting room, looking unobtrusive. He's taken his cap off, and he's placed a wicker basket on the bench beside him. He exchanges a few pleasantries with our secretary, speaking very quietly, as though he's worried about disturbing us.

In the consulting room, I'm putting the finishing touches to a hospitalisation form while at the same time listening attentively to the conversation that filters, only barely audibly, through the half-open door.

I don't recognise him, although I know I've seen his cat before. Stranded with my form, I can't consult the appointments book. So I listen. I listen as an old man tells his story, his and his cat's. The cat is twenty years old. He nearly died five months ago, but I saved him. Two months ago the old man brought him in to have him put down. And then took him home again. This time he thinks the old tomcat won't make it past Christmas. He's resigned to it, he's had him for longer than he ever thought he would, and he knows you can't stop the advance of age and illness. He wants to bury his pet at the bottom of the garden.

I'll play the innocent. Act as if I haven't heard anything. A quick look at the elderly cat's records and it all comes back to me. A nasty mammary tumour, cystic, enormous, that I'd punctured. Given the animal's age I'd ruled out surgery from the outset, thinking that with this procedure and a few palliative drugs he could still have a few comfortable weeks ahead of him. When the old man brought the cat back, the cyst hadn't formed again, but he had a bad case of gastro-enteritis. Nothing to do with the tumour, probably. He was dehydrated, slightly hypothermic, and he'd stopped eating, but I did tests to rule out kidney failure and tried a simple medical treatment. Which had worked perfectly.

And this time?

'So, Monsieur, what's wrong with the old boy?'

'Oh. You know ... it's the end.'

He speaks as quietly as he did in the waiting room. I lower my voice a little. He's not deaf. The old cat grumbles a bit, but consents to come on my lap. I'd started the consultation in my usual way, sitting on the examination table so as to encourage the animal out of its basket. Not holding or forcing it, just waiting for it to allow me to stroke it and to come to me naturally. It doesn't always work, but this time it was all purrs, no hesitation, nothing more to be said.

'The tumour's ruptured, some liquid has drained and there's been some bleeding, but it wasn't as big as the first time you know ...'

The old gentleman holds his cap in his hands, kneading it and rotating it between his fingers. The joints of his fingers are white, white from gripping so hard, waiting for my verdict. He juts his chin forward, his tongue discreetly pushing his dentures up and down. I don't say anything. I roll the cat over and stroke his front. The old tom relaxes, lets me tickle his chin. He has a nasty crater-shaped wound in the middle of his abdomen, near the navel. Three centimetres across, one or two deep, in the subcutaneous tissue. Around the wound the fur has been licked and licked until it lies flat. The wound is slack, or nearly, and there's no blood. A few signs of granulation tissue, new tissue formed during the healing process, probably worn away by the constant licking.

The cat purrs, the old gentleman tells me about his ravenous appetite, how he loves being stroked, how he spends all his time snoozing beside the stove. I don't say anything.

*

A long silence. The old gentleman is waiting for me to pass sentence, for me to say: 'This time we'll have to put him down.'

I take a deep breath. The old gentleman juts his chin out. His cap has stopped moving. His fingers are white, so very white.

'Right. Two injections, a couple of tins of cat food, and he can go home. I'll give you a bottle of antiseptic and him some antibiotics. He'll be around to see in the new year.'

The old gentleman's fingers are pink again. But he's still gripping his cap. He lets out an 'aaah' of surprise and relief. I hold his cat out to him.

Merry Christmas.

Liberation

'You see, her incontinence is getting worse and worse, doctor. Wherever she goes in the bar she leaves a trail of urine behind her, and it smells terrible and we spend all our time mopping it up, so we put her outside, but she's ten now and ...'

A great lump of a labrador, 40 kilos at least, suffering from spay incontinence that had started around a year after the operation. We'd tried every treatment, but in the end nothing had worked. Every now and then, her elderly owner would decide to have another go, and would agree to let us examine her again and prescribe something else. It never worked.

But putting her down because she was incontinent would be just plain stupid.

'It's my wife and daughter who have to clean up after her, I can't expect them to go on like that ... and it's just getting worse.'

We were all in the consulting room. The labrador was stretched out on the table, while we stood round her with our arms folded. The old man was hoping that ... that what?

That we'd agree to put her down?

That we'd find a miracle solution?

There would be no miracle. We knew what a nightmare it was keeping the café clean, with the dog wandering around between the customers as they had their lunch, the protests of the wife and the resignation of the husband.

In the end they left me to make the decision on my own, because it's a miserable business, and because you can't put a dog down just because she's incontinent.

Or perhaps you can.

*

He'd gone away wearing the wooden expression of people who make it a matter of pride not to cry.

Not in front of me.

Every time I walked past their café over the following week I felt a twinge of remorse for the dog that would always be stretched out in the middle of the road, dozing in the sunshine. You'd always have to swerve to avoid her.

Then one day I bumped into the old man's daughter in the village. She came straight over to me. And shook my hand.

'Had you heard my father died last week? On Wednesday?'

No, I hadn't. I offered her my condolences. I didn't know what to say. I'd seen him only two days earlier, on the Monday. I'm not old enough to be used to my clients dying.

She explained that he'd had a bad heart for many years. That he'd died peacefully.

That he hadn't been in any pain.

That once his dog had been put down, he'd been free to go.

That it had been a liberation.

Work experience

If you want to be a vet, you need to start asking the right questions in your early teens. For me the decision was already made. I was already en route and admiring the view. That's why nowadays I take a lot of trouble with my school students on work experience: I don't just show them the job, I show them the whole job. Warts and all. I sketch out scenarios, invite them to think about issues that at that age went completely over my head. Who else will tell these kids that even if they make the grade they might be on the wrong track?

Now I've honed a tried-and-tested speech for my work experience students. And I have a lot of them. We always have an initial meeting, a short interview of sorts, more like a briefing. They often come with their parents, but I much prefer the ones who call the surgery themselves rather than hiding behind mum or dad. I sit them down in one of the consulting rooms, usually in the evening around half past six. Since I imposed this more formal structure, I don't have a problem with the 'My Little Pony'-type work experience kids. Or not so much.

Work experience is usually a teenager's first encounter with the world of work. These fourteen- or fifteen-year-olds want to be vets, or at least to see what it's like. Or at the very least they want to avoid doing their work experience in a supermarket or office.

*

'All doors will be open to you, or nearly all: I'll come back to that. The aim of this work experience is to introduce you to the vet's profession, as it says in your agreement. You won't be allowed to actually do very much, but you can watch and be there. We'll try to explain as much as possible to you, during and after appointments. And on the drive between visits, always a good time.

'I know you think being a vet is a dream job. And yes, we vaccinate litters of puppies and kittens, we mend broken paws, we do dressings and injections. But we also clear up the mess after dogs with gastro-enteritis, we watch as animals get old and ill, we're there to put them down. Being a vet is a fantastic job, but it's a tough one too.

'You'll get the chance to see everything. When we go to the surgery for consultations, you'll come with us. I say "we" because I won't be the only vet you'll be with. My colleagues will be there too, and the nurses, and it's important that you should see all the different ways of approaching our work and theirs. So you'll be there when we operate in the operating theatre. You'll come to the kennels, to the treatment rooms, to farms and to stables. All I ask of you is to be discreet. You should wear "ordinary" clothes like the ones you're wearing today, we'll lend you a lab coat. You'll be able to touch the animals, but only when we say so: often the cats and dogs are very friendly, but here they're often frightened too. So they might not react the way you expect them to. If we tell you it's OK, go ahead: be careful but not fearful. Occasionally I'll tell you that I'd rather go without you.

'Some clients aren't easy to deal with, and with you there it would be even harder. And for instance when we put a cat or dog down, because it's in too much pain and we can't treat it, it's a very difficult time for the owners, and they often want me to be alone with them. But if I can, I'll try all the same to give you the chance to be there when I put an animal down. You can choose not to, as you can with anything else: I said you had access to everything, but that doesn't mean you have to do anything. If you don't want to, that's no problem.

'If you're lucky, you'll be able to watch a calving, or a caesarean section. There will be births and there will be deaths. There will be sick animals, and there will be animals that come in for vaccinations. You'll also see us doing a great deal of paperwork. We won't make you watch us signing cheques or chasing up unpaid bills, but you'll see that we spend quite a bit of time on these things. Every profession involves a lot of paperwork. We have mountains of it. Being a vet isn't just about treating animals. I'll try to make you aware of my role as business manager, and of the financial side of things. And don't worry: there'll be litters of puppies to vaccinate too.

'Any questions?'

*

Usually there aren't. Not before their work experience, not during it. So I prompt them. I try to do debriefs. Especially after putting an animal down. Yes, this is their first experience of the world of work. But it may also be their first experience of death, and of the pain that goes with it. No one emerges unscathed from witnessing the pain and tears of an adult who is losing their companion. Or from the absurd and brutal suddenness of death.

This is the reality of my job, of my practice. Other vets have different career paths, do different things. Some get up before dawn every day to inspect the carcasses of the animals that we're going to eat. Some are attached to the military. Some study wild animals and treat them, oversee the health and hygiene arrangements of factory farms, or carry out research in universities or pharmaceutical laboratories.

We're all vets.

L'Origine

When the man came in carrying his dog in his arms, semi-comatose, we pointed him straight away to the first treatment room.

The drip was already in place and we'd started resuscitation before we exchanged any words about the nature of the problem.

'She's my best hunting dog, doctor. There isn't a dog in the region with a keener sense of smell or finer instincts.'

She was remarkable, his dog. Not just that, she was intelligent, gentle and sweet-natured. Irreplaceable. Sadly she was also ten years old. Which for a hunting dog was long in the tooth. She'd never had pups. Or rather, her pups had always been stillborn. This time the man had chosen the best sire for one last try: having a litter at the age of ten was really pushing it.

'You have to save *l'origine*, you have to preserve the bloodline! I know her urea levels are high, I know her hunting days are over, but I can't let her pedigree die out just like that!

Fine.

Calculating from the date when she was covered, she had to be pretty much at full term. A quick scan to check: the pup was alive. For the mother things weren't so clear. Tests confirmed she was developing a serious metabolic complication, and that she needed to give birth very soon.

We scheduled the caesarean for the afternoon, which left us the morning to patch up the future mother.

By late morning she was in a coma, and we embarked on an emergency C-section. Without anaesthetic: she was no longer with us anyway.

Intensive care, help with breathing, the pup was born alive: it was a singleton, and it was enormous, which was why it had got stuck. A boy.

Our efforts had paid off and we could finish off the operation in the normal way: even the mother was saved, for the moment at least.

The man wept for joy.

The mother took almost 24 hours to come round completely, but her metabolic complications were less marked and she was lactating normally. The pup was in robust health.

Two days later, the mother's condition appeared to deteriorate. Metritis – inflammation of the uterus – and mastitis. We changed her antibiotics, put her on a drip, force-fed her; two days later, despite all our efforts, she died.

Since the infection started she'd had no milk, in any

case. We took turns to bottle-feed the pup, eight or ten times a day or even more – the nurse as she answered the telephone at the desk, any of the vets who happened to drop in on the ward between two appointments. The whiteboard filled up with little black crosses, each one of them signifying a feed.

My colleague ended up taking the pup home with him, so that his children could feed it when they came home from school. When he got it home he declared: 'We have to save *l'origine*.' And so, as they watched television, had their tea, in the evening, during the night, when the youngest had a nightmare, they saved the bloodline. Him, his wife and his two oldest children.

Thanks to all these exertions, the pup's growth curve eventually became normal.

It was exactly a week after the mother was admitted that we made the phone call: 'We've saved the pup, he can go home, but he's going to need a lot of looking after.'

When my colleague handed the man the pup his face lit up. His expression was priceless, especially when my colleague said:

'My children have looked after him a lot. They've found a name for him.'

The man looked at him questioningly.

'He's called *L'Origine*. And we've saved him.'

*

L'Origine has grown up into a magnificent hunting dog. All his mother's and father's qualities seem to have fallen by the wayside, on the other hand, but the old man isn't bothered. Now and again he reflects that qualities can jump a generation, and that with a stud dog and all the pups he'll be able to sire there's bound to be one good pup at least.

A bitch, perhaps.

Carnage

Saturday, 12 noon

It's very quiet when I go home for lunch. After lunch there are three appointments, really straightforward things, removing stitches and the like. For the past few weeks (months?), Saturday afternoons have been very quiet ... As I leave, a woman runs into the surgery carrying a cat. My colleague Olivier is on call, he'll take care of it.

Saturday, 14.05

I'm a little bit late. Olivier and Perrine, one of the nurses, are already there. As I pass the open door, Perrine calls out from the other side of the surgery:

'There are two hunting dogs with gashes from wild boar in the courtyard, and another one's on the way!'

Sigh.

Scarcely have I passed the doorway when a pick-up truck screeches to a halt behind me. It belongs to Benoît, a young local hunter. I can hear the unmistakable howls of wild boar hounds.

Tonight I'm invited for dinner with some friends. I haven't seen them for ages.

I don't even turn to look as Benoît gets his dog out of the truck. I head for the first two dogs in the courtyard. A quick glance reveals that one has its cheek slit open, revealing its jawbone, while the other has a very nasty bite on its upper hind leg, the muscles are torn but it doesn't look too deep. Both wag their tails when they see me at the kennel door. They can wait. I'll go and see the one that's just arrived.

Saturday, 14.10

Benoît is carrying the griffon and doesn't look too panic-stricken. I know him well, we have a good working relationship. He's a regular at the surgery, his dogs often get knocked about: they always tend to get in too close. When the boar stands its ground they should keep their distance. They've got attitude. That's what makes them good, says Benoît. This one looks pretty elderly.

I pull on my white coat.

'Was the hunt a long one?'

'Barely an hour, but they did a lot of running.'

'Quite old, this one?'

'Six.'

OK, drip to the max, it must be dehydrated, we need to protect its kidneys. I insert a catheter while keeping an eye on what's going on outside the door. Olivier quickly takes over the last appointment, and he'll be able to take care of the stitches too. Three dogs we can cope with. The telephone rings. I hear Perrine say:

'No problem, we'll be expecting you.'

Oh dear.

'More injured dogs, Benoît?'

'I dunno, they're all on their feet for the moment, I've just got these three.'

He holds the dog, which waits patiently and keeps still as I insert the catheter. It's soon asleep, and I give it a quick shave around the wound. I open box no. 1, small suture, and we stay in the prep room. The 'proper' operating theatre might be needed for more serious surgery.

Benoît looks worried. As soon as the patient is asleep, he dashes off after the rest of his dogs, which are still out hunting with his party. We clean up, disinfect, and I suture.

It's quite a nasty wound to the front left leg, a half-severed muscle, but it won't take too long to mend. Continuous suture to the muscle, insert drain, cutaneous suturing ...

Perrine pops in to see if I need anything, so I take the opportunity to ask her what's going on.

'What was the phone call about?'

'Another hunting party arriving with five dogs.'

Saturday, 14.45

Olivier puts his head round the prep room door, then goes off to finish the appointments.

I hear Perrine in reception:

'Could you weigh him please?'

Cyril, who hunts with another team, is standing in the

doorway, a dog in his arms. I'm busy finishing my suturing, and my patient is starting to get restless.

'What's the problem?'

'A small puncture under his stomach, with some fat coming out of it. And one of his pads is damaged, it's bleeding quite heavily.'

Indeed. The floor is red already, and the smell of disinfectant is being overwhelmed by the reek of blood. The small puncture wound is probably a rupture. The little bit of fat protruding will be part of the mesentery. Just as well – this is strong membranous tissue that's great for plugging this kind of wound. I've finished my initial suturing on the griffon, so I carry it to one of the cages.

'Put him straight on the operating table, I'm just coming.'

The bleeding from the paw doesn't seem too heavy, we'll look at it afterwards, it can't be too serious, I focus on the puncture wound to the abdomen. Catheter, drip, anaesthetic, the dog slumps, I put him on his back, the hunter waits for the diagnosis. I quickly shave a circle of about twenty centimetres around the little bit of fat that's dangling. I spend a few minutes cleaning it up and disinfecting it, then clamp it and widen the skin wound. A fine three-centimetre perforation right on the white line, I slip a finger into the abdomen, palpate the adjacent organs: liver, stomach, diaphragm, all perfectly smooth, no irregularities: an internal lesion is highly unlikely. I clean the bit of mesentery again and push it back into the abdomen. I'll insert a subcutaneous drain before I stitch it all up again.

Saturday, 15.00

I hear Olivier talking to one of Cyril's hunting party. Apparently one of the dogs has been badly injured. It's not putting its paw to the ground at all – a bad sign in these dogs that have an extraordinarily high pain threshold. If the dog can't put its weight on the paw it must be broken. Or worse.

A mobile rings: the hunters are sharing the latest bulletins. Olivier gives a rapid examination to another dog and announces a collapsed lung. On paper it's probably more urgent than the paw, but it's better if he does the paw as he's better at osteoarticular surgery, working on bones and joints, than I am. The collapsed lung can wait a bit in any case, and I've almost finished sewing my dog up again. I just need to have a look at his bleeding paw.

Saturday, 15.30

Olivier has put his dog under anaesthetic, and as he discovers the full extent of the damage to the humerus I hear him muttering 'bugger bugger bugger'.

I'm in the middle of examining the bleeding pad, while thinking ahead to the suturing of the collapsed lung that's coming next. The paw is more serious than I thought, the thorax and his collapsed lung will have to wait a bit: the wild boar has bitten between two pads and split them. And on top of that the wound is full of earth and sand. Cleaning, stitches ...

*

I hear the phone ring. Perrine answers:

'No problem. We'll expect you.'

Now I'm starting to hallucinate. I call her in, I need her to help me clean this injured paw in any case.

'What was that?'

'The Volp party, seven dogs at least, here in half an hour.'

Fifteen dogs between the two of us is madness. I ask her to call my wife, who's a vet but not working today, or not supposed to be at least. Otherwise there's no way we'll be able to cope. And I ask her to put off all appointments for the afternoon and to send any other hunting dogs to other practices. Fifteen dogs. It makes my head spin. I finish cleaning the dog's paw, extracting gravel, thorns and grass from deep under the pads. I'll stitch the top of the paw but leave an opening underneath. The hunter will have to clean it daily; it's pointless to seal it up hermetically as the wound is too septic.

I sigh:

'If any more hunters call in, tell them to go and see someone else.'

Rushing in with a pack of compresses, Perrine nods.

Saturday, 15.45

A hunter arrives at a run. Our third hunting party.

'He's got a neck wound, it's bleeding really badly!'

I do my last three stitches in a minute, then I tell Perrine to put the dog in a corner of the operating room so that we can keep an eye on it as it comes round. I tell the owner of the griffon with the wound to its thorax that he'll probably have to wait a while. The dog looks at me, wagging its tail, as I run out to the car park.

I return with the hunter, who carries his prostrated dog inside and lays it on the operating table. Perrine barely has time to give it a quick wipe. We're well past that stage.

While this is going on, I hear Olivier sighing as he assesses the damage to the shattered paw. Shredded muscles, scattered fragments of bone: he decides to do an X-ray. Listening to him, I wonder whether it's worth bothering. Hunters aren't that keen on three-legged dogs.

Working very quickly, I insert a venous catheter with a bag of colloids, to help restore blood volume; the dog is almost drained of blood but it's got a regular pulse and is breathing and conscious. Not for long, as the anaesthetic drugs – barely a quarter of the dose it should have in theory – send it to sleep. I put the dog on its back and stretch its head back. Its owner leans over it beside me, his anxiety palpable. I know him well, a Limousin breeder who I often see for his cattle. A friend, almost. I make no attempt to reassure him:

'The wound is in a really bad place, I'm afraid one of the branches of the arteries going up to the brain may be torn. Here it's blocked by a big clot, which is stopping the bleeding. But there's a danger it will begin again as soon as I start to explore the wound. It might finish the dog off, but we don't have a choice.'

I hesitate. If I leave the clot where it is and simply close up the wound it might work in the short term, but in a few days there's a danger that the clot that has stopped the haemorrhage might disappear before the artery has healed up, which would mean another haemorrhage and probably the death of the dog. Also, I don't really know the extent of the damage that lies beneath, and the larynx is only a few millimetres away. I decide on the interventionist approach: if the dog dies, at least I'll have tried everything. Working very slowly, I start to dissect the torn muscles, gradually going in deeper towards the hyoid apparatus, and the carotid arteries. I'm not too confident. It could all blow up in my face at any moment, spraying blood everywhere.

Saturday, 16.20

One by one, I separate the multitude of muscles that criss-cross this small area of the throat. Where does this one go? Up or down? I advance methodically, gradually removing the fragments of blood clot, expecting a haemorrhage at any moment. It's getting deeper and deeper, and I'm beginning to wonder just how far the wild boar has penetrated. I begin to worry about the windpipe. The dog hasn't spat any blood, so it shouldn't be damaged? But the hunter might have missed it in his panic. He's just told me that he found another of his dogs beside this one with its throat slit, dead. He's white as a sheet.

Unsure, I put my instruments aside and insert my fingers at the base of the dog's throat, palpating and examining. The haematoma is visible through the pharynx wall, but I can't feel any tear. Hesitating, I intubate the dog, which will help me to locate anatomical structures as I dissect.

As I continue my tentative exploration, I discover a new disaster: the hyoid apparatus is broken clean through. The function of these tiny bones is to support the larynx, pharynx and tongue: without this, I'm not sure whether the dog will be able to swallow or breathe normally. It's impossible to repair the bone, it's just too delicate. The wound doesn't appear to go much deeper. Underneath it, I find a torn 'small' artery. It might have bled a lot, but it's much less serious than a carotid, it's OK. I close it all up, attempt to stitch the muscles around the hyoid apparatus, then close everything up, one layer at a time. I explain my doubts and fears to the dog's owner. He'll have to keep it on a liquid diet for several days and make sure it avoids any strain on its respiratory system. It may not be able to swallow. The hunter takes it well: he trusts me, and that hurts; I feel so small in the face of all this damage. I finish the stitches. The collapsed lung is waiting in the corridor. I'd almost forgotten about it, and about the eight or ten other dogs all waiting to be patched up. I hope my wife will get here soon.

Saturday, 17.00
The dog with the throat wound is in a cage in the kennels, with a drip and blankets.

The next hunter has already put his collapsed lung case on the operating table. Is he fed up with missing his turn?

I turn to the dog and give it a quick examination. The heartbeat is impeccable, I can hear the characteristic sound of air between the pleurae, one of the ribs is broken. For the time being, the hole is more or less plugged by the muscles and skin. I take my time getting everything ready. Insert a catheter and drip, choose an endotracheal tube and prepare the anaesthesia circuit. While I do this I explain to a hunter standing beside me how to use an anaesthesia breathing bag on a dog. I hope my wife will be here soon.

Olivier delivers a loud commentary on his X-ray for my benefit: bone fragments all over the place but there doesn't appear to be any serious damage to the bone, so he sets about stitching it up.

The telephone rings. When Perrine informs me that Monsieur Dupont is waiting for us to take bloods from his ewe I can barely conceal my irritation. I speak very loudly for his benefit.

'Tell him that we're very sorry but it's carnage here today and we can't come. It's not urgent, so he'll just have to make another appointment for next week.'

She nods, then joins in the game, repeating the same thing in a slightly more roundabout way. Then she hangs up.

'He's cross.'

'Too bad, if he's not happy he can go somewhere else. Anyway, he always gets in a huff when we don't run around after him.'

The telephone rings again. I heave another sigh. Perrine rolls her eyes.

'No, we can't do it, we already have three packs of dogs here.'

Standing there holding the anaesthetic gel for the endotracheal tube, my white coat covered in blood, I have difficulty getting my head around it. Four packs. She hangs up.

'It's Roque's team, they've got four injured dogs.'

She hesitates: they weren't happy.

Too bad, they'll understand.

I hear my wife's voice. She's arrived and is taking in the scale of the disaster. I follow her gaze. The floor is a shambles of blood, shit and mud from the hunters' boots, with trails of footsteps where we've tramped through it all. There are at least seven hunters now, reliving the day together, watching their dogs anxiously, listening to my explanations or keeping an eye on the latest dog to come round. Some have gone outside, sickened by the blood. Others are itching to join in when I palpate a wound and describe the damage.

Blood is sprayed all up the walls from the dog with the collapsed lung on the operating table: as it quietly pants for breath it carries on wagging its bleeding tail. With those war wounds. Dumb dog.

Saturday, 17.45

I anaesthetise the collapsed lung case, placing the dog on its back and intubating it; it's not fully asleep and I have to wait. My wife has put on a white coat and is attempting to get a handle on this scene of chaos. We insert the endotracheal tube together as I fill her in on the quirks of our anaesthesia circuit. Perrine dashes from room to room, keeping an eye on things, replenishing stocks of compresses, and fetching catheters, transfusion bags and more reels of suture material. 'She must have covered a few kilometres by now', quips one of the hunters.

After shaving, cleaning and disinfecting all round the wound to the thorax, I make a broad incision in the skin in order to get a better view of the damage to the thoracic wall. There's a broken rib, the opening is wide enough. I stitch the intercostal muscles, a continuous suture that I'll close up at the last minute. Next door, I hear Olivier exclaim:

'It's not splinters of bone, it's bits of wild boar teeth!'

The hunters crowd in to see. Meanwhile, on our side of the wall, I reach the end of my continuous suture and my wife checks the breathing bag. The fateful moment arrives: in order to re-establish the vacuum in the pleural cavity, we'll have to inflate the dog's lungs with the breathing bag, compress its abdomen, and close the stitches – all at once.

'Perrine, I need a hand! Now!'

She's close by and she knows what to do: my wife compresses the bag, Perrine compresses the abdomen, and I tighten my knot.

Merde! All of a sudden the dog's skin swells on the side of the thoracic wall, fifteen centimetres from my suture. Two holes!

'Double pneumothorax! Drop everything!'

I make an incision in the skin to discover the second wound: a second broken rib, nowhere near the first one. I put the finishing touches to my first suture. When the second one is ready we'll go through the same process all over again.

Next door, in a low voice, Olivier is explaining to the owner of the dog with the injured paw that he's repaired the damage but that it will need a lot of physiotherapy. If there's no nerve damage. In which case it will have to be amputated.

Saturday, 18.00
My second suture is ready, my wife and Perrine are back in position, the dog's owner is watching.

'OK, we'll restore the vacuum. On a count of three!'

Total silence, we all wait for the dog to start breathing on its own again, while keeping an eye open for any small leak from the suture. One. I redo a stitch, then spread the wound in order to start the process of re-establishing the pleural vacuum.

'One. Two. Three!' I tighten the knot.

Silence again. No leak this time. We all get back to work. My wife offers to finish the cutaneous suture, and there's a lot of work to be done. One or two drains, a star-shaped incision. I agree. I'll be more useful assessing the injuries of the other dogs. Micro-surgery is more her thing.

Olivier has already started on another suture, for a wound to a joint.

The hunter has gone outside for a smoke.

Saturday, 18.15
As I head for the consulting room, I talk to the hunters of the three different parties. I leave it up to them to decide who'll be seen next. They suggest two different dogs, I

choose a wound to the thorax. The hole is small, but it might be deep: another collapsed lung? I notice another dog with the same type of wound: perhaps a third. Luckily the first one doesn't really need help with breathing any more. We'll see soon enough.

I wash my hands with antibacterial soap, the Gascon hound is on the operating table, wagging its tail. I tell the hunter that I'm going to examine the wound and warn him that he'll need to hold the dog. I insert my fingers into the wound, feeling for the passage to the pleural cavity. The dog whines a little and wags its tail harder. There probably isn't a collapsed lung. I decide to anaesthetise it: it will all need stitching and a drain in any case.

Perrine comes in and asks what I've done in each case, keeping a record for the accounts. While I insert the catheter and anaesthetise the dog I tell her, adding the antibiotics, anti-inflammatories and other opioids used on each of them, as well as the follow-up prescriptions they'll need afterwards.

I've lost track of what's going on at the back of the surgery, in the operating theatre and the prep room, but it hardly matters. I insert a drain, do a muscular continuous suture, a subcutaneous continuous suture, a cutaneous continuous suture. On to the next one. Benoît, one of the youngest of the hunters, comes round with a bag of sweets, unwraps them for us and stuffs them in our mouths while reading out the little printed quotations enclosed in the wrappers, his great boots squelching through the puddles of blood smeared around the floor by the oozing mop.

Saturday, 19.00

Another blue griffon with a wound to the thorax is brought in to me. I dare to hope that my findings will be the same as with the last one. There's a small wound to the sternum as well. Someone tells me that Olivier has finished the articular suture:

'He's stitched the, erm ... joint capsule.'

'If he doesn't get osteoarthritis or even arthritis your dog will be lucky.'

As I examine the wound and anaesthetise the dog I talk to the hunters. This is definitely not a collapsed lung, but a major cutaneous and subcutaneous tear. Some simple stitching and a drain. With all the dogs, the reek of dogs and blood and wild boar, the hunters chatting with each other and calling their friends and families ('We'll be late back') – with all this activity, at once frenetic and laid-back, the atmosphere in the surgery is extraordinary. All around there are discussions about the weight of the wild boar involved, the length of their tusks, and the different injuries produced by females' teeth and the males' snouts.

Saturday, 19.30

I call the friends we're supposed to be having supper with tonight. We're going to be late.

Now people start to bring me dogs with very superficial cuts. A few staples and a stitch on the sternum and groin of the first one, a bitch. She doesn't appreciate it, but the hunters hold her securely. It's not the first time for her and she doesn't cry, even though she doesn't seem very keen on my needles. Perrine tells me that my wife is repairing an eyelid, and Olivier is stitching some masseter muscles in a dog's jaw.

I move on to the next dog, a simple cutaneous suture and a small drain, with just a few minutes of anaesthetic this time. I'm on automatic pilot. Olivier comes to ask my advice on the next dog. I can tell he's flagging: under normal circumstances he wouldn't have asked for my help in such a case. Our brains may be turning to mush, but our hands still know what they're doing. At least I think they do. I search for my catheter. Where can I have put it?

Saturday, 20.15

My wife is done, and is now checking a dressing on the two-hole case. Olivier is finishing off an awkward wound in the middle of a dog's neck, before anaesthetising the last one. The last one, really and truly. I take a deep breath. That's it, it's over. I stretch my spine, my back's sore from bending over the tables. Benoît eyes me with a gently mocking look, bag of sweets in hand:

'There's one left if you want it?'

A bitch arrives, hopping on three legs.

I lift her on to the table, give her a quick examination, anaesthetise her. The wound is near the knee and it's deep: my metal probe penetrates over fifteen centimetres between the layers of muscle. It will need a drain.

Cyril, one of the hunters, puts his head round the door of the consulting room, now transformed into the antechamber to a horror film:

'You haven't told me about treatments for Athos and Uno?'

And I hear a voice ask:

'Doctor, do we need to wash the drain?'

My wife offers to finish off the knee surgery. I grab my prescription pad and blister packs of antibiotics. For one dog after another, I explain the dressings, post-operative care and check-up visits that will be needed. I write it all down. I reiterate my fears for the dog with the damaged hyoid.

I heave a sigh. It's nine o'clock.

At half past nine, we set off on the hour-long drive to our friends. It will take Perrine and Olivier another hour at least to do an initial clean-up and keep an eye on the most traumatised dogs as they come round from the anaesthetic.

Time for our out-of-hours service to begin.

Choke

It's eight in the morning. The calf is nestling in a cow-shed in the crook of a valley. I finish inserting a catheter into his ear. The day started too early, but at least this one should make it. A drip for the day, or the morning at least, and with a bit of luck he'll be out enjoying the sunshine that the forecast has promised us.

My mobile makes a vague bleeping noise. A text message. At this time in the morning it will be someone wanting to make an appointment. Normally I don't answer calls, I filter them. But this time I couldn't have answered anyway: any time you get mobile coverage round here it's strictly only by accident. Occasionally something will go wrong and a text will get through. Orange covers 99 per cent of France; I'm one of the thousands who live in the remaining 1 per cent. I check anyway: 'You have four new voicemails.'

Damn.

Voicemails aren't about appointments. Voicemails are about emergencies. I finish inserting the drip, lob out anti-biotics and the rest, scribble a prescription and sprint up the nearest hill, where I should get a signal.

Success. The voicemail is from nearly half an hour ago. And it's a genuine emergency. The message is hysterical, but it's nothing compared with the ones that follow. A horse with choke, an oesophageal obstruction, from swallowing alfalfa granules too quickly. The horse is calm, she says. *She* isn't, though. Not remotely by the time she leaves her fourth message. I don't even listen to it. Have I got everything I need in the car? Parked half on the verge and half on the country lane, I inspect the contents of the boot. Silicone nasogastric tubes, paraffin oil, red catheters, anti-spasmodics, antibiotics, anti-inflammatories. But I haven't got the pump, or the anti-tetanus serum.

I'll have to make a detour via the surgery. In all, it will take me a good half-hour to get there. Meanwhile, the surgery is open now and taking calls so I don't have to. A quick dash into the supply store to grab the pump, and a serum from the fridge. I take another bottle of analgesics, just in case, and I know I have sedatives. And a bag of bran mash.

As I leave, the first nurse arrives. I ask her to call Madame Dussans to let her know I'm on my way. No point in leaving her to stress unnecessarily.

*

I'm coming, but it's a long way. I detest choke. A horse that's a bit greedy and a big dose of bad luck, and a blockage of granules can form in the oesophagus, often at the entrance to the thorax. The horse coughs and coughs, and there's a high risk of food 'going down the wrong way' and being aspirated into the trachea, and of lesions to the oesophagus. My last two cases of choke ended very badly. So it goes without saying that I was already pretty tense, especially as the owner of this horse is a long way from being the easiest of customers. I always have a problem working with people who are under stress, hard to please and – because it goes with the territory – aggressive in their attitude. If everything goes according to plan, they simply take it for granted. If it doesn't, it's an absolute scandal. So I do my best to batten down the hatches and just focus on the animal, which has as much right as any other to the best possible care. But I know I'm not as good. I don't have the temperament of some of my louder colleagues, who have the knack of shutting up clients when they seem to be trying to win some kind of prize for being thoroughly disagreeable.

*

I park near the loose box. The woman is with her horse, her dogs and her husband. She is calm and smiling. So is he. Has the horse managed to void the obstruction?

Sadly not.

I guess I should stop making mountains out of molehills.

The horse appears calm too. No straining to cough, no obvious nasal discharge.

I load all my paraphernalia into the toolbox. A quick auscultation: I'm listening above all to the breathing in the trachea and as it leaves the nostrils. The chestnut gelding's warm breath caresses my ears. There's moisture and a little bubbling, but nothing serious. The trachea is dry, but you can hear the pain in the arytenoid cartilages. I disinfect around the jugular, shave, insert the catheter. I've got the time to do the job properly. An injection of anti-inflammatories to deal with the pain. I test the nostrils with my finger. Korn (seriously, who'd call their horse Korn?) doesn't like it, any more than most horses like having a vet's finger stuck up their nose. Sedation. I've got a catheter in place, so I might as well make the most of it.

Two minutes later the sedatives have done their job, and Korn's muzzle is stretched out flat on the floor. I start to investigate his nostrils with my largest nasogastric tube. I'm taking a bit of a chance, as he's not that big, but if I can manage to insert this one the lavage, or flushing out, will be easier. My first attempt fails, and I'm in the trachea. It was bound to happen, as his head was really stretched too far back. But we're not here to practise neck extensions with Koko, so I ask Madame Dussans and her husband to draw his head in behind the vertical. As he's under sedation the horse allows them to move his head, and between them they struggle to hold it in the position I need. This time I get stuck. A good sign. I ask them to move the head to the left a little, to the right, down a bit, and at last I can get past and into the oesophagus. I'm making progress. They can let go of the head.

The horse coughs once, and evacuates a great stream of saliva through his nose.

I stop straight away. The marks I made on the tube have rubbed off already. Too bad. I must be there, just at the entrance to the thorax. Nothing comes out spontaneously.

I pump in a little warm water. The horse doesn't complain and keeps his head low – my preferred configuration in this type of situation. If liquid rises back up the oesophagus, as it nearly always does, it won't go down the trachea.

A little more water, I withdraw the tube by five centimetres, then push it back in again. Still nothing. I wait a little, to allow the water to loosen the obstruction. Back down goes the tube, another two or three centimetres. A little more water again. This time, green liquid starts to seep down the tube. With difficulty. It's very thick. I draw the tube back and launch another attack, send in a little more water. This time it overflows, and alfalfa trickles out of Korn's nostrils. Not much of it, and he doesn't move. That's OK. I carry on chipping away, slowly, gently, forwards, backwards, never forcing, never injecting too much water. I suck on it but it doesn't help, and a mouthful of horse saliva and alfalfa isn't that tempting a prospect ...

We'll get there. Between the effluvia emerging via the tube and via the nostrils, in the end it will be enough. I'm squatting down over Korn's right nostril, fiddling with the tube. Monsieur Dussans is crouching beside me, ready to hold the tube in position when I go to operate the pump.

The horse is completely knocked out by the sedative. He doesn't make any attempt to raise his head, which helps the partially dissolved granules to flow out. The green liquid oozes gently down the tube. A little more water.

I push the tube deeper, twisting it gently on itself. I can see that Korn is starting to get restless. Still sitting beside me, Monsieur Dussans strokes the horse's cheek. Here I am, my green heavy-duty overalls pulled on over my T-shirt, squatting on a hillside, in the entrance to a loose box, enjoying the sunshine for which we've been waiting for weeks now. Monsieur Dussans is beside me, still crouching down, his green dungarees half open.

Korn shakes his head to left and right. Then quickly raises it for a moment and without any warning gives a sneeze. The accumulation of alfalfa and saliva in his nostrils shoots out in two great plumes. The left-hand one hits Monsieur Dussans' neck, spot on. The right-hand one hits mine. We're both covered in mucus, saliva and alfalfa. Madame Dussans fails to suppress a laugh.

It feels ... tepid.

*

A quick sluice down in the bucket of water and I carry on with the job. I'm a bit more wary now, though. A quick dive to my left and I manage to avoid the next sneeze altogether. Not so Monsieur Dussans. My eyebrows are drying out, the hairs all stuck together. This time I think that's it. I insert the tube a bit further, give a little push, go deeper. I'm not quite sure how we're doing, so I go back to the pump. The water flows in, no problem. Another go, then a third: this time I know it's reaching the stomach. I draw the tube halfway up the oesophagus, wait a little, then remove it completely.

It's over. I listen to the lungs again. I can't hear anything untoward, but the heartbeat is so loud that I can't be completely sure. The trachea is still dry. The larynx is less painful. This time it's all good.

An antibiotic, a few words of advice.

By the time I get back to the surgery it's eleven o'clock. Time to start the morning's work.

Ending a life

It's a moment like no other. For me it's always the same, a moment when I swallow hard and accept a choice, our choice: the choice made by the animal's owner and by me.

*

'Right. Before we start, I need to explain briefly what's going to happen. But first of all you need to know that you can choose whether to stay or to leave. The nurse can help me, you can wait in the waiting room, or you can stay with us. You can be on your way home. Or you can hold your pet. I'll shave a patch on her paw with a razor. That might scare her a little, but I need to do this in order to insert the catheter. This will be the only difficult part for her. Once this flexible plastic needle is inserted in a vein, I'll be able to anaesthetise her. It will be a proper anaesthetic. She'll be unconscious in no time at all, probably before I've even finished the injection. It will be so quick that there won't be any feelings of nausea or disorientation: she won't even be aware of it.

'It's a real anaesthetic. She'll be in a very deep sleep: I could operate on her and she wouldn't feel a thing.'

Her owner nods.

'When she's in a deep sleep, I'll be able to give her the second injection. This will deepen her sleep into a coma, and it will paralyse her breathing, and then her heart.'

*

The owner may stay, or they may choose not to. It's easier for me if they go, naturally. But of course it's completely fine if they decide to stay.

Most owners give their pet a last cuddle while I go off to fetch my tourniquet, alcohol, two catheters, some sticking plaster, and the anaesthetic and euthanasia drugs. On the way to the room where these are kept, I signal to the nurses: euthanasia in progress, do not disturb on any account.

I often feel a bit wobbly. Or else I'm panting like an ox. It all depends on how the consultation that led to the decision went. Did they come with this in mind? Is it the culmination of a long-drawn-out series of treatments? Is this the outcome we expected, or is it the result of some brutal accident? Have I had to negotiate to avoid it happening earlier? Or, on the contrary, have I had to raise the subject?

As I go to fetch the drugs, the time for all these considerations has run out. And yet. It hasn't been difficult to set up a process that suits us all for making this type of decision. All the vets who work here reserve the right to refuse to put an animal down. Our reasons for doing so would be more or less the same, and we wouldn't put down a dog if one of our colleagues had refused to do so.

Unjustified requests to have an animal put down are rare. But they're spectacular. We've experienced slammed doors, raised voices, and spluttering objections: 'But he's going into a home and we can't look after his dog!' We've experienced accusations and threats. And we've experienced clients who have stalked out, declaring, 'Well, if it's like that I'll go to a different vet. He'll put him down!'

Yeah, right.

And then there are the clients who try to manipulate us. We're aware of this, to a greater or lesser extent. And with all this, we have to make the decision. To put them down or not? If you refuse, what would be your reasons, and what would you hope to achieve? You have to bear the animal's interests in mind, but you shouldn't use them as an excuse to avoid a difficult decision. If the owner can't keep an animal any longer, it can go to a rescue centre or home. Most people can't bear to admit that their pet can have a life without them.

*

I go back to the consulting room. The owner's eyes are red. The animal is waiting, usually very patiently, at the limits of its endurance. It's asleep. It's anxious, blind, deaf, disabled; it's unable to understand what's happening to it, as it can neither hear nor see, and it's aware only of that worrying smell of the vet's surgery and of its owner's distress. So many people feel that they are betraying their companion. And in a sense they are. And me? I'm here to heal, not to kill. But ...

If all goes 'well', this will be an 'easy' euthanasia. Sometimes I won't be able to insert the catheter because the animal is too dehydrated or panicky. In such cases the injection has to be done into the muscle. I don't like doing it this way. It's too slow, too unpredictable. But often I don't have the choice. There's an alternative method I can use, a mask and gas. Keeping the mask in place isn't always easy though.

The second and final injection has to be delivered intravenously. There's no choice in the matter. If there isn't a vein, it has to be done directly into the heart.

'I'm so sorry, I can't do this injection intravenously as I can't find a vein. I'll have to do it another way, which might be rather upsetting. I'm bound to explain to you what's involved, but you don't have to watch. He's asleep, and he can't feel anything at all; I'm going to inject the drug directly into his heart. Death will be instantaneous.'

*

I hate it when I have to do this. It's too easy to get it wrong and to inject into the pericardium. And then the animal still feels nothing, granted, but death is far from instantaneous. The drug takes minutes to circulate, and it seems interminable. And then it's so, well, violent.

But my clients are never so grateful as they are when I have put their pet down. Of course people are grateful when I manage to treat a disease or operate on their dog. Sometimes for treatments that are extremely complex and impressive. Sometimes for minor things that are frankly completely routine.

But when I've put their pets down, they send me cards, letters, sometimes even little gifts.

'*Merci, docteur, merci.*'

But ... I've just killed their cat, I've just killed their dog.

Light as a feather

It was a few days before Christmas when he arrived with us.

So frail and fragile that we didn't dare touch him, for fear of hurting him.

Winnie the nineteen-year-old Siamese cat. Nineteen long years.

Winnie wouldn't eat, was slightly dehydrated, and if he did manage to swallow the odd scrap of food, promptly vomited it up again.

He seemed so light, light as a feather – a feather of grey fur with black markings, a touch unkempt, with a few clumps of matted fur, a touch unsteady on his paws.

He was standing on the edge of the table, hesitating, wobbling, teetering, not daring to jump. His mistress stroked him, drew him back to safety; there's no way he'd have been able to stop himself from falling.

I thought his old kidneys had finally failed. I'd started to prepare his mistress. But Winnie didn't have high levels of urea. Winnie had diabetes.

Who would ever have imagined that at nineteen his diabetes might be treatable?

Was there any hope of stabilising him?

A small tumour, a failing pancreas or a chronic inflammation that we'd never suspected, who knew what might be at the root of it? It scarcely mattered: too much sugar in the blood, not enough in the muscles, too much in the brain and the urine, a metabolism that was completely out of kilter because insulin wasn't being secreted as it should be.

It would take several days to get him back in balance. To adjust his doses, check and verify them, feed him, hydrate him, transfuse him and stroke him.

To be there for him.

His family were due to go away in a few days, for Christmas. And despite the nineteen years they had shared with him, they couldn't change their arrangements.

Winnie would be spending Christmas at the surgery. On the ward. Cuddled, fussed over, looked after, but on the ward.

They knew there was a chance he might not be there when they got back.

It was the 23rd; they'd be back in five days, on the 28th.

By then he might be dead.

So Winnie stayed behind. The treatment was working a bit, not enough, and crucially he wouldn't eat. He was in better balance, Christmas was coming, and Winnie stayed on.

All alone in his cage. If there weren't any call-outs on Christmas Day, I might not go to the surgery at all.

So it was purely and simply to avoid making a few return trips for his treatment and tests that I took him home with me. Obviously. It was past nine o'clock when I went into the bedroom. What a festive way to spend Christmas Eve. I had a basket, a bottle of insulin in an insulated bag, a few needles and syringes, a blood sugar meter, and Winnie.

My wife felt him rubbing himself against her hand, light as a feather, as the weary old cat tiptoed his way up the duvet and settled down to sleep. Much to the chagrin, the total outrage, of our two resident cats.

And then we stroked him.

Fussed over him.

Looked after him.

Hydrated him.

And tried to get him to eat, but to no avail.

Not diabetic cat food, anyway. Not any cat food, full stop.

Home-made wild boar pâté, on the other hand? Now that was a different kettle of fish.

Just the once: after that he wasn't interested.

The next day it was foie gras, no less. Just the once.

Then scrambled egg.

Grilled chicken.

Smoked salmon.

One laboriously chewed mouthful at a time, swallowed with difficulty. And only ever just the once.

The aromas of pâté, foie gras, salmon and eggs lingered on in the bedroom, but he'd lost interest.

His diabetes was getting into better balance. I was coming and going to work.

He stayed at home, on our bed, almost until the end of the holidays, until his mistress came back. I delivered him back to her, advising her to tempt him with all the treats we hadn't yet tried. Winnie was leaving, lighter than ever, purring, pampered, but dying.

He died two days later, in the bosom of his family.

And the diabetes? In balance ... but at nineteen it was too much to hope for more.

But he'd tiptoed up my duvet, light as a feather.

He'd stretched out there.

He'd purred.

Boots off

It's Sunday morning, half past six. An old farmhouse perched on a hillside, an old-fashioned cowshed, four cows no longer in their first flush, a small herd of sheep and a retired farmer and his wife.

The cowshed is clean, with wholesome aromas of cows, straw and hay, hens in the manger, a Border collie on a hay bale and a red Massey Ferguson tractor that's older than me.

The front door to the house is reserved for Sunday best (if then, even); on other days the way in is through the cowshed, where a couple of steps under the stairs up to the hayloft take you straight into the kitchen.

The old farmer, a tall and rangy Clint Eastwood looka-like in beret and braces, has called me out because his cow is dilated, and she's turning round and round in circles, but nothing's happening.

'You're an early riser!', I'd remarked when he called.

'*Mais non*, I've been up all night with her!'

'Ouch. In that case you go to bed late! In any case, I'm on my way.'

He hadn't called me earlier because, well, it was the middle of the night, but now that he'd waited he was afraid he might have put the calf's life at risk.

*

The cow is a big blonde. Huge. Laid back. Placid as a Volvo estate. With a boot capacious enough to accommodate the most outsize of calves.

I pull on my overalls and gloves and go out of the rain and into the cowshed. He pulls the stable door shut, first the bottom and then the top, and we position the cow facing it. One arm in. Her waters aren't broken, I can feel a front leg. A nice calf. I grope around a bit and find the other front leg, then the head. Facing down. And, crucially, a textbook uterine torsion. The uterus and vagina have twisted through 180 degrees, and however hard the cow strains the calf won't pass through the birth canal, as the tissues can't dilate far enough. The calf is alive, but as usual I say nothing – especially as I haven't been asked.

I'd heard the door to the kitchen as it opened behind me. Madame has closed it behind her and is standing on the bottom step, waiting. She's wearing the dress and pinafore that look so right on her but that only she can carry off, the sort of dress and pinafore that are like a uniform, so natural that you take them for granted. You could poke fun at Monsieur, in his beret, braces and checked shirt. You could poke fun at Madame, with her little glasses on a string round her neck and her print dress. But if anyone dared to laugh at them I think I might whack them in the chops with the metal pulley of my calving jack. I feel so comfortable here, in this little cowshed, my arms in the birth canal of a blonde cow, wisps of straw in my hair, in the warm, with this old couple, while outside it's raining.

You have to rotate clockwise. Positioning my right arm is easier, but I lack sufficient strength and it's breaking my wrist. The left arm then, my back to the cow almost, and a major twist from the shoulder to the spine: yes, but my wrist's still breaking. Still, in this position I have more traction. Left arm, then right arm again, little by little, steadily. The calf is still in the amniotic sac, and I know I'll get there in the end. I swap sides, pushing, turning, moving round. Gradually, barely five minutes in, I find the right rhythm, the right impetus, syncopated this time. My left wrist hurts. The ribs on my right side are pulling, tight across my back.

The calf is facing in the right direction again. I breathe a little more easily.

We've got time.

*

Everything is in place. Monsieur is setting up the jack, Madame has gone to get a saucepan full of water. Stainless steel, not copper. My resuscitation box is here, with my caesarean equipment, which won't be needed. I've got my calving ropes. The cow starts to paw the hay again.

I could stop there and go home: she doesn't need me any more. But the farmer wouldn't understand why I'd left, for one thing. I'd be chewing my nails not knowing if I had been right to leave, for another. And for a third, I want to get this calf out.

So I plunge both arms back in up to the shoulders. Warm, slippery, comfortable, with that sweet, sickly smell of amniotic fluid. It feels good. Just the place to be at seven o'clock on a Sunday morning. Outside, the sun is rising after the rain. The Border collie stirs on its bale of hay. One leg, two legs. I grasp them firmly, draw them towards me; the mother strains a little. Everything is in place for the birth. It's a big calf, but there's room for it. The mother's waters have broken now: the fluid gushes down my overalls and over my boots into the straw that fills the gutters. It's all good.

Now the second sac, of that thick, runny mucus, of that indefinable white colour, from which life flows.

I draw the feet towards me, the head follows gently, the baby's forehead gets stuck against the pelvis. It will come, we just need to give it a little pull.

Madame brings me the ropes, my good old stout calving ropes that have been bleached and put through the wash hundreds of times. I position them around the calf's cannon bones, well above the fetlocks, and I lean back, my body almost horizontal, shifting my weight first to the right then to the left, my feet wedged in the gutter. The calf is so strong that it manages to pull me up by retracting its left foreleg. My weight against its weight, my supports against its supports. But I'm not plastered all over with calving mucus, or not as much as it is, and I've done this before.

The cow is well dilated. The farmer took his time before

calling me, so there's no danger of an episiotomy, of having to make a surgical incision.

It's all good.

We attach the jack. The cow lies down, exactly as she's supposed to. Monsieur pulls, Madame takes care of the ropes, while I guide the 'baby' as it comes into the world. In absolute strength and power, a gentle violence. And absolute confidence.

The little creature is now fully out, much to her amazement. Lying in the central passage, she breathes in and out, a bit dazed. Still lying down, her mother is calling her already. A little water behind the ears, a deep breath in, a noisy breath out, lots of mucus. As a precaution, we'll hang her upside down. She's spent a long time upside down inside her mother. I knot a rope around her hocks, Monsieur sends Madame to fetch a chair so we can pass the rope over one of the beams. I remove some mucus from the calf's mouth with my hand.

Madame positions the chair.

Monsieur stops to take off his boots, then climbs up on to the chair. Brushes away a few spiders, passes the rope over the beam. I lift up the bouncing baby, all 50 kilos or so of her. He gets down, checks his grip and takes a few steps backwards. Mucus pours out of the calf's nostrils. She's breathing well, we lower her again. I guide her as she lands on a mattress of straw. The farmer picks up his pitchfork and scatters some straw over her back to keep her warm.

We get the mother into a standing position, and I pull gloves on again to check that nothing is torn.

It's all good.

*

'Would you like a coffee?'

'Oh yes please, but first I must take some photos. They're for, erm ... for my sister – she just loves pictures of baby animals. Silly really, isn't it?'

'Oh, if I'd known I wouldn't have put the straw over her!'

He smiles.

I click away.

You can be 75 years old and still appreciate a moment like this.

Then afterwards, yes, we'll have a coffee. But before I climb the two steps up to the kitchen, before I cross the threshold, there's one thing I must remember to do, above all else, before all else. I must remember to take my boots off. Even if he protests that there's no need. And I know he will.

Chronic kidney disease

I don't know if anyone's ever told you just how vile a thing chronic renal disease is.

I'm not talking about acute, sudden kidney failure that can be brought on by some other illness, which if treated generally means the kidneys can carry on with their essential work of filtering and purifying our blood.

No, I'm thinking of chronic renal failure, the 'natural death' that awaits so many cats and dogs, the failure of the most fragile of all their organs, their hope for life. With us it's our arteries that fail, or our brain. With them it's their kidneys.

There's a sort of wear-and-tear threshold, at around 25 to 30 per cent of the initial renal capacity, when the kidneys start to seriously struggle to do their job, although the animal isn't necessarily really ill. You can detect it by testing the urine, or sometimes the blood. Occasionally you can detect it before it gets a hold. Then often you're in with a chance.

In many cases it's diagnosed only because renal failure has really set in: the kidneys aren't working properly, waste products are building up, and uremic syndrome is beginning, with all its many repercussions. We try doing transfusions to force the kidneys to filter out impurities. This can work, and work well, if the kidneys still have some capacity. If they have been plunged into crisis by an accident of some kind, there's hope for getting the system working again. And then there are some animals that survive very well and for a long time with creatinine or urea levels that should by rights have killed them. As usual, it's a case of treating the animals, not the test results.

But when the end comes it's horrible. An ugly, long-drawn-out death. It's not the heart that gives out, it's a slow descent into auto-intoxication. It's not for nothing that we put so many pets down. We'd all rather they died in their baskets, in their sleep.

Number 2298

Number 2298 is eighteen years old.

Number 2298 is just an ordinary cow.

Number 2298 is generally good-natured, but neither more nor less so than other cows.

Number 2298 is an elderly cow with a vague resemblance to a Blonde d'Aquitaine crossed with who knows what.

Number 2298 is still with her herd, despite her age, because she's always lived a placid life and has calved every year and fed her calves without any problem. And also because she can still get about. She just happens to have outlived the usual age for being put out to grass by six years.

Number 2298 fell over on her side a few weeks ago. She couldn't get back up again. The farmer got her up on her sternum, wedged her with a hay bale, gave her some water and called me.

Number 2298 was four months pregnant and crippled with arthritis. I gave her an anti-inflammatory injection and advised the farmer to use straps or a crowbar to get her back on her feet so as not to leave her lying down for too long, and to make sure she ate, especially hay, and drank.

Number 2298 was up on her feet within a few hours, and went back to her daily routine.

Number 2298 fell on her side again a few days ago. She couldn't get back up again. The farmer got her up on her sternum, wedged her with a hay bale, gave her some water and called me.

Number 2298 is a bit thin, but only a bit. She's still in fine fettle, she has no detectable neurological deficit, she still ruminates, but her temperature is slowly going down. She's weary. Weary of carrying her calf, which hasn't yet begun the rapid growth phase of the last months of gestation. Weary of clambering up on to her feet every morning, weary of her haunches that won't do what she wants any more. I give her an anti-inflammatory injection, but there's not much advice I can give to the farmer. He's already done it all, even clearing out the stall, leaving just a thin layer of manure to help her get a grip on the beaten earth below. Number 2298 just can't really support her own weight any more.

Number 2298 didn't get back up again, despite the farmer's efforts. Two days later, he called me out again.

Number 2298 was lying on her side. She'd pushed away the bales of hay that were keeping her lying upright. She still looked in reasonable shape, she was still eating and drinking. The farmer came with me, a fixed expression on his face. His father chose to stay behind in the farmhouse.

Number 2298 is dead. I put her down.

Number 2298 lived eighteen good years, with no major incidents. She gave birth to sixteen calves, some of which have bred further generations in their turn. Three, four, five generations? Others have gone to the slaughterhouse.

Number 2298 was born when the farmer was a small boy. He saw her being born and helped her give birth to all her calves, guided their first steps, sometimes helped them on to the udder. He took them to their mother to suckle, morning and evening. He looked after them, watched them grow, watched them go.

Number 2298. The farmer was her lifelong companion, from birth to death. In her last days he devoted himself to her care. He got her back up on her feet, turned her over to avoid pressure sores, fed her, took the time to give her water, spread out her mattress of straw, cleaned up after her. He asked me to do what I could for her and he didn't quibble over the cost of the anti-inflammatories, even though he knew that her last pregnancy would never reach full term.

'I owed her that much at least', he said.

Number 2298 was a nondescript old cow, one of those old cows that have been bred out now. The pride of the meadows. She died in about 30 seconds, with no pain.

Number 2298 was just an ordinary cow. I killed her.

Number 2298 was eighteen years old.

Putrefaction

A WORD OF CAUTION: *This chapter contains a scene that some readers may find upsetting. My editor wanted me to take it out but I insisted on keeping it in. Firstly because anyone who knows anything about what a vet does would be surprised not to read about scenes such as this. And secondly because I don't want to endorse any misconceived idea that vets spend all their time cuddling adorable puppies. Happily this type of event doesn't happen very often, but to be a vet you have to have a strong stomach. Those of a sensitive disposition might be advised to skip this chapter and turn to page 112.*

It's half past eight in the evening, an injured labrador has just arrived at the surgery, and the phone's ringing again.

'I've just got back to the farm and found one of my ewes can't get up. She had a lamb yesterday morning. Do you think there might be another one left inside her?'

Not likely. But not impossible either. I hesitate as I tell him to come and pick up some antibiotics, anti-inflammatories and a little sugar and calcium, because ... well, he might just as well bring the ewe in with him, didn't he think?

Whatever happens, I've still got work to do on my lab-rador. The drip's in place, the anaesthetic's done, the dog's stabilised, the X-rays are ready. A shattered tibia. I finish off a dressing to support the wound in preparation for trans-ferring him tomorrow to colleagues who can operate on him. It only takes about ten minutes in the end, but I still have to look in on my in-patients, check the till, prepare the handover notes and send in the order. And while I'm at it I might as well expand some over-succinct consult-ation notes.

I've got nothing else to do while I wait for my ewe to arrive, anyway.

I've even got the syringes prepared. When she gets here I'll bung in a thermometer, find out if there's an infection, give her the injections, and we can all go home.

*

The guy has parked his C15 van outside the entrance, its rear doors facing the surgery door to take advantage of the light. It's only a couple of hours since the place was cleaned: no way is the sheep coming inside.

The ewe is lying on her side. She can lift her head and she looks alert.

'She can't stand up. I had a real job getting her into the van.'

Yeah, very sorry, but I had to look after a dog that had been run over, it would have taken too long for me to get to you, and in any case this has saved you paying the price of a call-out. Agreed?

A solid 80 kilos of sheep, I can well believe she wasn't easy to carry. She's had lambs four times, twins every time, and this time it was a singleton. Not surprising that he should think there might be a second one left behind. Temperature of 39.2, heart beating faster than normal, but then after that journey ... Mucous membranes OK.

In any case, there's nothing like a good feel along the birth canal with your arm. Even into the uterus. There, at the far end, is a sac, almost a perfect sphere. Through the membrane I can feel bones – there's a lamb in there all right. I try to grasp a bone – a shoulder blade? – through the membrane, but it doesn't respond. Dead, clearly. The sac is strange, granular. Chronic placentitis, an inflammation of the placenta? I'm surprised she's still alive. I'm even more surprised that I can't puncture the sac. Anyway, with my gloves on it's hard to know what I'm feeling. I think I can make out the spine. The lamb must have presented curled up with its back first and got stuck like that. There's no question of taking my gloves off, though.

I've switched to mouth breathing – an automatic survival mechanism for vets.

The ewe puts up pretty well with my investigations and manipulations. She strains without any effect, but she doesn't struggle too much. I slide my hand and arm over the dorsal face of the uterus, to feel all around the lamb and work out its exact position. Oh look, the membrane's thinner here. I try to puncture it.

And I'm not disappointed: out flows a flood of foul-smelling gases and blood-streaked matter with a stench of well-hung game, all streaming out of the back of the van and into the surgery doorway.

A hoof.

The farmer is standing ten or so metres off, looking nauseous.

The lamb is putrefied, its body swollen with gases, and what I took for a malformed foetal sac was in fact its skin, blown out from its body by the gases of putrefaction. The thinner area was the skin of the abdomen, under the stifle joint in the hind leg. Now I can feel the skeleton and muscles better. Its head is facing down towards the ewe's udder, with a leg to each side probably. That's where I'll have to set to work.

But first, antibiotics, anti-inflammatories, intravenous drip.

This time I slide my arm over the ventral face of the uterus. It's much less easy because of the curve. I've got my gloves on, naturally, but I know they won't be enough and my hands will stink of decaying flesh for at least 24 hours. As for my jumper, the less said the better. As I crouch on my knees at the back of the van at nine o'clock at night, in the dark and the rain, I conjure up mental visions of midwives in hospitals, with state-of-the-art delivery suites, birthing pools and childish decorations in pastel palettes. In my dreams.

Locating the nape of the neck, I slide my fingers to either side of the lamb's head. It's all slithery, I can't get a hold. The jaw slides away. I try to grasp the front leg from above, and manage to do so without too much difficulty. I draw it into the pelvic passage, then I turn the head. This will mean I can raise the lamb up a little, which will make me feel I'm making headway.

The next stage goes on for another ten minutes or so. Try to get a grip on the head, straighten it and pass it through the pelvis. No way. It catches on something every time and slips out of my grip. Even though I've found some fingerholds. There's the jaw: too fragile and also dislocated. Or the eye sockets: not bad, but you'd need to have bloody strong fingers to use them to pull the head up. And just imagine the stomach-churning sensation of the eyeballs as they explode between your fingers. Or the neck: yeah well, OK, but the angle's never quite right.

The ewe, meanwhile, has given up. She's not moving any more, but her breathing's good. She's in pain. In shock.

The stench is atrocious. It's the stench of the knacker's yard, of a dog that's rolled in rotting flesh, of clots of black blood and gobs of putrescence, splattered all over the ground and all over the van. As I manoeuvre the lamb I do my best not to get it all over my trousers. In that respect I don't do too badly.

I don't know what I've done right, but eventually the head appears. In a tragic state, but in the right position. All I have to do now is to jam my fingers in one more time to straighten the other front leg, and the final extraction will be a mere formality. I pull out the lamb's body, and the farmer begins to realise just how hellish it was inside. The body ends up in a dustbin bag, with a trail of putrid blood polluting everything as it passes.

I still have to fix up a drip for the mother, otherwise all this will have been for nothing. Corticosteroids and analgesics. The farmer asks if she'll pull through. I've no idea, but I think so, if the uterus is intact. Every twist and movement, every attempt to lever up the limbs, skull and body of the lamb had to be done without putting any pressure on a uterus that has inevitably been weakened by infection. If it's been punctured, the ewe is done for. If not ... we'll see tomorrow. I don't give him any medication: he can come back and get the drugs tomorrow, if there's any point.

As for me, if I don't want my clients passing out when they arrive in the morning I've got to swab down the surgery doorway. And the hose isn't working. So I fetch the bucket, the long-handled scrubbing brush and the bleach. It's not even raining hard enough to help.

It's a quarter to ten, just about time to go home.

Sexplousse

There he was, sitting on the other side of the desk. Olivier was in his chair, I was leaning in the doorway. He hadn't touched his cup of tea yet, and he seemed a little awkward, with his little laptop displaying great Excel spreadsheets and his neat piles of papers, carefully arranged and rearranged.

He couldn't leave them alone: he kept picking them up, tapping them up and down to straighten them, then with immense care putting them back in their piles in front of him. He was wearing a three-piece suit and tie, he didn't have a hair out of place, and his watch was a good one. Not the usual look for the drug company reps sent to beguile us with the latest products or tempt us with miraculous (they were always miraculous) business contracts.

Olivier had greeted him with a cheery 'Hello, Monsieur De Mesmaeker!', a witty reference to the popular French comic-strip character of a wealthy businessman who's forever on the verge of gaining a lucrative contract but never quite does so.

The reference went over his head, as it had with all the others. He corrected Olivier politely:

'Oh no, I'm Benoît Laroche, you must be confusing me with my predecessor, I'm the Sexplousse rep for this area.'

As usual, we welcomed him politely, and after a bit Olivier stopped making remarks along the lines of 'So have you got the contracts, Monsieur De Mesmaeker?'

Anyway.

The Sexplousse drug company sells one product and one only, a treatment for arthritis. It's been selling this product for some twenty years. Maybe thirty. Maybe longer. No one's ever really understood how it worked, nor indeed if it worked, but as you can't ever be sure, and occasionally it has appeared to work, many vets have continued to use it. It can't do any harm, in any case.

As usual, the rep was about to present us with a new study offering infallible proof of how effective this product was, and as usual we weren't going to buy any of it.

As usual, we were wondering how we were going to say 'no' without being rude. He wouldn't last long in the job, just as his predecessors hadn't. For lack of results, I imagine.

*

Now he was off. He looked as if he was revving up, ready to launch into his spiel, and we'd been making idiotic jokes so as to give him a chance.

'The cell membrane is an ocean of lipids with icebergs of proteins floating in it —'

We couldn't help it. We didn't actually burst out laughing, but we couldn't stop ourselves from gawping at him in disbelief. You see, that sentence is the ultimate tired old cliché in any description of the cell membrane, the one that all our teachers and professors at school and vet school would invariably trot out sooner or later. And there were pages of the stuff to go!

So we stopped him.

Clearly he didn't understand a word of what he was spouting. So we got him talking about his product, about the business opportunities, anything but that lecture on the phospholipid bilayer. We tried to get him to relax, to help him to understand:

'You see that spiel of yours, it's so elementary, we were spoon-fed it for two years, maybe longer ...'

His 'business opportunity' was a lot of hot air too (but it went without saying that we weren't going to buy large quantities of this stuff, so there wasn't a lot he could do).

Then one thing led to another, and we found ourselves chatting. Sitting there in his pink tie, three-piece suit and improbably neat hair, he was now fighting back the tears. Because we were nice to him, he said, where other vets had sent him packing, jeering at his product for being outdated and at him for being shy and incompetent. We explained to him why no one was remotely interested in his product. And why they were even less interested in studies that were largely a load of hogwash. There wasn't a vet in the area who hadn't made their mind up about it ages ago.

So then he told us. In his previous career he'd been a rep for luxury products, doing the rounds of smart hairdressers and beauty salons. He liked it, but then the firm he worked for went out of business.

So he ended up applying to Sexplousse for a job.

He hadn't realised it was a lab making veterinary pharmaceuticals.

Sexplousse.

He thought it was a company selling sex toys.

What's a life worth?

It's a difficult subject. A subject that gets people hot under the collar, that we prefer to avoid, churning out stock responses, not stopping to think. *Life is worth the price we put on it. An animal is just a possession. You can't put a price on a life.*

It's a subject we try to ignore.

Because … 'when it comes to my dog, money doesn't come into it, he's my playmate, my cuddly toy, my faithful confidant, my beloved companion – not like my boyfriend, who walked out on me.'

Because … 'my cat lies on my bed in the morning and purrs, and he has such funny annoying little ways when he wants to be fed.'

What would you say, though, if I told you that your cat had cancer, and that I could offer you two alternative courses of treatment?

Let's say that the first treatment is highly effective, with very few side-effects, and could give your cat another six months to three years of pain-free life. It will require very close monitoring, and will cost around 2,500 euros. A course of chemotherapy.

Only six months, maybe three years?

*

Or else you could opt for a simple cortisone treatment, which will probably slow down the spread of the cancer and allow him to live comfortably for another three to nine months, at a cost of around 30 euros.

Only three to nine months?

*

Which one would you choose?

*

Or would you avoid the question, like so many people, and with it the question of cost?

'Oh no, not chemotherapy, that's awful, I wouldn't put my pet through that!'

Or would you protest that the money isn't important? This is almost never true. Of course the money is important. Of course it's important to know how much it will cost. Of course it matters, because the times when owners can treat their pets without counting the cost are vanishingly rare.

Perhaps you would ask how much a course of chemotherapy for your cat would cost after six months? To which I would reply 1,200 euros. And then you might calculate that cortisone will also give him six months of comfortable life, but for 30 euros. We'd talk about the survival rate, the chances of his surviving another year, or two years. You'd probably tell yourself that when it comes down to it cortisone isn't so bad. You'd reflect that there are people who don't even have access to polio and tetanus vaccinations, which cost just a few euros. And you'd be right. But you'd also be haggling over the life of your cat. And what would you think if, despite the very best care, despite the 900 euros you'd already paid, your cat died five weeks into the treatment?

Or else you'd tell me that you can't afford to pay 2,500 euros for your cat, even over three years. You'd be ashamed. You'd blame yourself. And I'd feel the same, because I wouldn't be able to offer you the treatment for less. Because in fact 2,500 euros for a course of chemo-therapy isn't expensive. Does that shock you?

Me too.

We're talking about how much you'd be prepared to pay for your pet's health. About how much its life is worth.

*

Some clients protest that 65 euros for a vaccination for a perfectly healthy cat is expensive. Yes, I agree: 65 euros for an animal could be described as a luxury, even. It's also a basic necessity, however, if you want to protect it against fatal diseases such as panleukopenia and leukaemia. Not to mention the value of the consultation for a vaccination, the number of points I check, the symptoms I might pick up on. A vaccination isn't just an injection. So yes, it's worth 65 euros.

*

How do you define the value of a life?

Its monetary value is the cost of the animal. There aren't many people who are prepared to pay for treatment for their child's hamster that cost 8 euros.

'You can just buy another one. And it'll teach the boy about life and death. And it costs 25 euros for a vet's appointment! And even if they find something there'll be nothing they can do.'

Then there's the emotional value of a life, the amount these same owners would be prepared to pay to have their pet treated. How much would that small boy have paid to save his hamster? Everything he had, probably.

But in real life it's all so much more complicated. Vets deal with people from so many different social and cultural backgrounds. I tried to define my clientele for one of my work experience students, so he could put it in his report:

'It's geographical. This is a rural area, and my clients are the people who live within a twenty-kilometre radius. They include small farmers, hunters, manual workers, doctors, well-off people, poor people, children, men and women, old people, a priest, and a home for people with disabilities.'

And all these people relate to their animals in their own individual way. To their own animals, and to other people's.

I know one woman of retirement age and pious views who deplores the way wild boar hunters send their hunting dogs out in the full knowledge that they'll take a beating. So I tell her about those dogs, dogs that would do anything – even when mortally injured – to get back to the chase, dogs that just love to hunt. Dogs that are miserable when they see the pack going off without them, leaving them behind just because they're a mass of stitches.

I also know a very old lady who could never get used to the idea that she could enjoy such little luxuries as care for her pet, no questions asked. That day she was paying 50 euros or so to have her cat neutered. Some 60 years earlier, during the war, she had fled Lille in the north of France, which was occupied by the Nazis, to reach the unoccupied zone in the south. According to her own private logic, now she was lucky to be able to spend 50 euros on her pet.

Then there's the practical use to which an animal can be put.

It might help its owner to earn a living, like a sheepdog or a guard dog. It might help them to live with a disability, like a guide dog. It might bring them in an income when it's sold, like a Limousin calf (probably their only source of income). Or it might provide them with a leisure activity, like a hunting dog or a gymkhana pony. Or – most likely – it might have no real 'use' whatsoever, like your cat. Yet it has a value.

And then there's the status we give our pets, their social standing, if you like.

For some people a dog is just a dog, however much they love it. They're happy to pay, as long as the amount is 'reasonable'. To some people in rural areas, a cat is little better than a weasel, virtually vermin. 'Who'd buy a cat? Some people are mad.' Other people will pay a lawyer to negotiate custody of the Yorkie that their ex took with them when they left. How will the lawyer explain to them that in law a dog is merely a possession? And most people fall somewhere between the two extremes, the happy medium. Happy? Happy for whom, exactly?

Then there's the length of time an animal can be expected to live.

Who would pay thousands of euros to give their sixteen-year-old dog another month of life? Lots of my clients decide to stop having their dogs vaccinated when they reach a certain age, when in fact the protection vaccinations offer is even more important at an advanced age. Some refuse to treat a broken paw because the dog is old. Others don't care how old the dog is and feel it's the least they can do. A cattle farmer won't spend a lot of money on an elderly cow that can no longer produce milk or calves. He'll send her for slaughter. Who's right? Who's wrong?

Lastly, there's how much we love our animals, purely and simply. You never ask yourself the question, but one day I might have to: how much are you prepared to pay? I sincerely hope it never happens to you. But the question's an interesting one, all the same. And a chilling one. Probably not one you want to ask yourself.

So why would you answer it on anyone else's behalf?

*

A car driver runs over a dog. It wasn't his fault, he was driving at normal speed and the dog ran out in front of the car. How much should he be prepared to pay to treat its injuries? Or the dog's owner, if the driver has driven off? Or what if the driver finds out that the dog is a stray and no one will miss it? How much should the driver pay if this time it was his fault? If he tells himself that it could have been his own dog? If he tells himself that it could have been a child?

*

A farmer asks the vet to put down one of his cows. How much extra is it worth to spare her suffering, rather than just letting her die, which would cost nothing? The cost of her vaccinations and the price of her calves?

And when we buy a steak, how much are we prepared to pay to ensure that the animal is slaughtered painlessly? According to opinion polls, we're happy to pay extra. People are so generous. Yet often in fact they buy the meat that's cheapest, rather than meat from countries where abattoirs and animal suffering are strictly regulated.

Each one of us places a different value on the lives of animals, a value that is shaped by all these considerations, both rational and irrational. So before we judge others we should try to understand them. It's what I have to do every day.

At the same time it's not my decision, though: I can offer alternatives, and I can make adjustments to suit different clients. The little boy who's weeping inconsolably over his rat will pay a token amount, but he'll still pay. As a token, precisely. The woman who wakes up every vet in the area in the middle of the night to have her cat spayed as an emergency will doubtless be charged more than someone else who makes an appointment in the normal way. Most of the time, happily, I only have to give estimates, perhaps offer different ways to pay, and leave the owner to wrestle with their conscience.

*

And you, what preconceived notions do you have?

Do you think that because a farmer sends his cows for slaughter he doesn't care about them, that he'll pay as little as possible for any treatment and certainly won't indulge in anything that isn't strictly necessary? You might also remind yourself that he spends his life up to his ankles in manure and doing backbreaking work. That he's subject to regulations governing animal welfare and health and hygiene that you have no idea about. And on a small farm, how much return does he see for all his work, in the end? Maybe he doesn't do it for the money. They play the hard man, as I know only too well, but they share their lives with their animals. I'd like you to see one of these callous brutes when I have to put one of their animals down.

And what makes you think that those loutish hunters don't care about their dogs? You'd be surprised to know how much they spend on feeding them, hunting with them and looking after them. And how much time they spend training them. You should see their faces when one of them falls by the wayside.

Is a dog with a pedigree as long as your arm, say a Shar-Pei that cost 2,000 euros, worth more than a cross-breed? Of course not. So why is this charming and kind owner prepared to lavish so much money on her new pedigree puppy, when she's just had her old 57-varieties mongrel put down, even though it could have been treated?

What is the value, in rural France, of a goose bred to be force-fed for foie gras? Would it shock you to know that one of my clients paid 2,000 euros for a triple osteotomy operation on a seven-month-old Bernese mountain dog? Why do horses that have worked at the equestrian centre get sent to the abattoir rather than being put out to grass? What price would you put on the life of a Rottweiler that displays threatening behaviour, growls at people, and has already bitten someone?

How much?

Why?

Odour of vanilla

Monsieur and Madame Hermann are a retired couple in their early seventies.

For the past nineteen years they have shared their lives with Gitane, a highly-strung little five-kilo ball of fluff, whose state of health you can imagine only too well.

An appointment with Monsieur and Madame Hermann has something of a ritual about it.

First of all there's the image that meets my gaze as I open the consulting room door. They make a perfect couple. Monsieur Hermann wears a black coat, a fine burgundy-coloured jersey and a grey scarf. His thick silvery hair is immaculately cut. He has a grey hat, and his black shoes are impeccably polished. Madame Hermann wears a fur coat and a discreet toque, a silk scarf knotted at her throat and a floral gilt brooch pinned to her breast. There's nothing self-conscious about their appearance, nothing showy.

Close on the heels of this image comes the scent, the vanilla notes of Madame Hermann's perfume, heavy and insistent, almost oppressive. Curiously, it's this perfume that sets the all-pervasive, overriding tone in all my encounters with Monsieur and Madame Hermann.

Not Monsieur's voice, deep, calm and steady, nor Madame's more anxious tones.

Not Monsieur's handshake, firm, supple and restrained, nor Madame's brush of the hand, light and almost imperceptible.

Instead it's that odour of vanilla, the scent that also clings to the fur of Gitane, who now lies trembling in the arms of her mistress.

*

It's the third time this year that Monsieur and Madame Hermann have brought Gitane in to see me. Gitane is nineteen. Like all lapdogs of her advanced years, she has a heart condition. She's almost blind with cataracts. But otherwise she hasn't lost her faculties, she's not disorientated, and her reactions are perfectly normal.

Madame Hermann could tell you more about her than I can, if only she could stop referring to her in the past tense.

'She used to be so lovely, such a dainty little fairy with her golden curls, and so intelligent, so affectionate. Such a darling!'

These days Gitane isn't so lovely, but you could still say that she looks good for her age. Her coat is very fine, but dense and soft. Her skin is flawless. She's beautifully turned out. Her joints and postures are normal. In short, she's not one of those drooling elderly dogs that you hesitate to make a fuss of, and only do it because you remember when they looked good and didn't smell bad.

Four months ago, we operated on Gitane to remove a mammary tumour. It all went well, despite the risks of the anaesthetic, and the wound has healed nicely.

Monsieur and Madame Hermann have brought Gitane in today because she has a sort of scab on her right eye, which is oozing slightly and covers the lower lid and a few square centimetres of the skin below it. It's clearly troubling her, and Madame Hermann struggles to keep it clean. My first thought, like hers, is that it's an accumulation of a mucous discharge from the tear ducts, complicated by a skin infection.

Using tiny scissors and a minuscule scalpel blade, I start to lift off the scab, millimetre by millimetre, all the while avoiding the snapping teeth of a little dog that is evidently in a lot of pain.

Eventually I discover that this oozing scab doesn't come from the eye, but from a small hole in the nasal wall, an infraorbital fistula, a classic complication of a sinus infection, itself caused by an abscess on a tooth. Gitane's teeth are in a catastrophic state, obviously, but until now we haven't wanted to run the risk of giving her an anaesthetic in order to scale them.

But now we have no choice. As long as there's a rotten tooth behind it, this lesion has no chance of healing, and antibiotics alone won't be enough to tackle an infection like this. The treatment will have to be surgical: extraction of the rotten teeth and scaling of the rest, followed by anti-inflammatories and antibiotics. The anaesthetic will probably be quite long and the operation will be painful. The risks of the anaesthetic will be very high.

But we have to treat the dog. We can't leave Gitane in so much pain. She's had these dental abscesses for some time, and the drugs she's been given haven't managed to check the infection. Her pain threshold must be high, but there are limits to what we can expect her to endure. Madame Hermann confirms my suspicions: she's barely eating any more, and she often rubs her muzzle on the ground.

*

'So we have to accept the risks of the anaesthetic if we want to allow Gitane to carry on with a decent quality of life.'

I deliberately to phrase it like this in order to leave the way open for her owners to broach the subject of putting her down. Gitane is nineteen, she's in pain, the surgery will be painful, and she has lots of other things that are starting to go wrong. If they decide they want to put her down, I won't refuse. They get my meaning.

'If she dies during the anaesthetic, would she suffer?' Monsieur Hermann's voice is grave.

'No, she wouldn't suffer. And at least we would have tried, rather than merely resigning ourselves.'

Madame Hermann gives her husband a look of agreement. She asks me if I think the operation will really help Gitane, which I do. So she chooses surgery, and rejects euthanasia. After doing a blood test, with excellent results,

I prescribe some medication and make an appointment for the following week.

That night I have a nagging feeling that something's not right.

*

It's a week later by the time I put my finger on it. I'm checking Gitane in for her operation, and by the time I put the little dog in her cage, Monsieur and Madame Hermann have already left. The odour of vanilla is oppressive. I wonder ... I wonder whether they aren't actually hoping that Gitane will die under the anaesthetic. Consciously or otherwise. Like that, they wouldn't have had to take the responsibility of putting her down, and they would have done everything they could for her, for this companion who has shared nineteen years of their lives, for this little ball of fluff that used to be so lovely. Such a darling!

There's a leaden feeling in the pit of my stomach. What if I were to give her just a little too much anaesthetic? Just a fraction?

She wouldn't suffer.

They would be relieved, their consciences would be clear.

And nobody would know.

I toy with the idea for a few minutes. The odour of vanilla is all-pervasive.

I don't tell a soul.

*

Three hours later, very slowly, Gitane comes round from the anaesthetic. She's on morphine and completely disorientated. In a little basin are ten rotten teeth. Everything has gone like clockwork.

In the afternoon, Monsieur and Madame Hermann come to see her.

As they leave, I shake their hands. We'll keep Gitane for today to control the pain. She can go home tomorrow.

A few minutes earlier, as they were on their way to the kennels with one of the other vets, I'd heard the uneasy note in my colleague's voice:

'But she's still lovely! She's dribbling a bit just for the moment, and there's some blood, and she's dazed by the morphine, but tomorrow you'll have your little Gitane back!'

I could just imagine Madame Hermann murmuring, 'But she used to be so lovely!'

As the door closes behind the two of them, I turn to look at my colleague, standing hands on hips at the end of the passage. She looks rattled. Fragile. Lovely.

'When I told them everything had gone well they seemed ... disappointed.'

I shut my eyes. Just for a moment.

Medical vocabulary

A small cowshed, an elderly couple, their daughter and their granddaughter. Six years old, confident and inquisitive.

I start on a caesarean, a once-in-a-decade operation on this farm. On a cow that they've just bought, a pseudo-Parthenaise heifer that – to judge by the size of the calf's cannon bones – must have been crossed with a Charolais.

I didn't even try to pull, but just got ready to operate, nice and relaxed. There was no great urgency, mega baby was nice and cosy where he was. I'd only have the old boy to help me pull, but still, that shouldn't be too much of a problem. He spends his days mucking out the cowshed and shifting bales of hay: he might be elderly, but he's undoubtedly stronger than I am.

The heifer's a little bit skittish, but not too bad. A few ropes, a local anaesthetic, and it'll all be done and dusted. I shave the animal's flank. A single cut.

Everything's ready now.

A long vertical incision, the hide and then the muscles parting under my blade. An arteriole sprays me scarlet; in the cowshed silence reigns. As I puncture the final membrane, the peritoneum, air rushes into the abdomen with the sound of a toilet flushing.

'Mummy, does it hurt?'

'No, look, she's not even moving, she's not crying.'

I investigate the abdomen, get my bearings. The calf is huge. It reminds me of my early years in practice, when I used to do C-sections in the Charolais region. Uterine incision. I grasp the back hooves and turn the uterus, lining up the uterine incision with the abdominal incision. The two hooves, red with blood, are now pointing in the direction of the outside world. The old boy attaches the ropes and starts to pull. I help him by lifting the hocks, but the hindquarters refuse to pass. Our efforts become increasingly frenzied. I grab my scalpel, enlarge the abdominal opening. Still no good. One more go with the scalpel, this time it's bound to come. I can see the tendons standing taut in the farmer's neck, I'm pulling with all my might, sweating, the effort is so violent, so extreme that I'm almost tempted to give up and drop everything, and bloody hell the damn calf just won't come out, it's just sitting there, with the umbilical cord stretched tight, half in half out, its head stuck in the amniotic fluid, it'll be curtains if we don't get it out really soon, if it breathes in it'll drown, it *will* breathe in, it'll *have* to, the cord's compressed, its ribcage is still inside, the old boy can't take any more. *PUTAIN DE BORDEL DE MERDE DE BITE A CHIER DE MERDE DE PUTE DE VEAU!!*

It's out.

I'm pretty sure I let out a yell.

I've torn my biceps.

It's alive, it's breathing, I fall back on my heels and exhale deeply, whistling under my breath. The bucket of antiseptic is sitting in front of me: I duck my head into it, then gulp down half a litre of water.

Shreds of uterus and placenta are hanging from the cow's flank.

It's all OK.

'Mummy?'

'Yes darling?'

'What did the vet say?'

'Medical words. Words that you only ever say during caesareans.'

Mémé

The rain was lashing down, a vertical downpour like the pillars of a frozen mausoleum. A drenching, freezing deluge, blotting out the sombre winter sky and extinguishing all hope.

I was there on my own, quite alone. Why did I have to be on my own?

Standing there in the field, fists clenched, I called her, I ran and skidded about looking for her, but I already knew. She'd fallen down again. I cried, screamed and raged, opened the boot, grabbed the syringe and the bottle, put them back again. I'd spotted her, lying there, hobbled, tangled up in the straps of her blanket until I undid them. I paused a moment – I shouldn't have – to pull on my boots. Then I knelt down. Her laboured breaths would have formed little clouds, but for the freezing, stabbing rain. She lay there, drenched.

How many times before had we got her back up on her feet? How many times had we been convinced it was for the last time? How many times had we known that we were kidding ourselves? That we were wallowing in the pleasure of lying to ourselves, of living in denial? This time,

I wept. Great stifled sobs. I went back to the car to get the bottle, then turned round again. Went back one more time. I wanted to put it off. I knew that this time there was no more room for hope. Just cold certainty. I was soaked through. In a fury. In love.

So I went back again, and I knelt down beside her. I took her adorable great scrawny head of a useless bony old mare, the head that always used to wobble above her skinny neck and twisted legs, and I held it. Caked with grime, soaked through with rain, smeared with freezing, clinging mud, I took her great knackered head on my lap, stroking her, holding her, calling her name. She shut those great big eyes of an old mare, accepting the fussing and stroking that she'd always disdained in her old age. She was trembling. She'd fought and struggled, and I'd only just found her. Because I just happened to drop by to see her on my way to work.

I think I talked to her the whole time. With her head on my knees I filled the syringe, furious, desperate, overwhelmed by love and by hate. I was there for her, I tucked her in, I held her. She closed her eyes, sighing, letting me. Keeping her bony head in my lap, I leaned over her, applying pressure with my left hand, injecting her with my right.

'It'll be OK, Mémé, it'll be OK, old girl.'

Of course it'll be OK.

She gave a shudder, a tremor, then she died, there in my lap, my old bat of an old mare, my most beloved pain in the neck. She died in my lap, and I killed her.

I've never regretted it.

It was years ago now, and I still miss her. I'm so glad.

The awkward bugger
of a case

Sometimes you can spot an awkward bugger of a case a mile off, when a client says an animal is 'not quite right' or 'a bit off colour'. But often it can strike without warning. It may erupt as an emergency, it may emerge when least expected during a routine consultation, or it may even blow up out of a simple vaccination.

The awkward bugger of a case is a familiar companion, known affectionately to me as an ABC. But to my colleagues they're known as OFSs: Ones For Sylvain. They lob them in my direction, every time: I may not be a particular fan of surgery, but I do like a tricky diagnosis.

An awkward bugger of a case is a complex thing: a wide-ranging diagnosis with many possible trails to follow up and investigate. A good ABC will feature lengthy waits for test results, or expensive examinations, or preferably both. In a really good ABC the initial test results will be ambiguous, necessitating further investigation. Or better still, the results will clearly favour one hypothesis that you duly rush to embrace, only to be forced to abandon it again when further tests reveal possible alternative interpretations of the initial one.

When you try to explain an ABC to a dog's owner, simply and in layman's terms, in no time at all you find yourself tied up in a web of comparisons and metaphors that are so convoluted that you get everyone hopelessly confused, yourself included.

By definition, an ABC appears serious, but sometimes it's just an illness that's unpleasant and difficult to manage. Dermatology is the preferred field for this type of ABC. And as complex as these cases may be, in the end they can wear you down and chip away at your motivation. Because you just can't pin it down, somehow.

You can deconstruct an ABC visually on a large whiteboard. You can add loads of arrows and hypotheses, you can cross some out and you can add others on. It always terrifies my colleagues when I do this.

An ABC stands a good chance of being expensive, and if it requires multiple examinations or a stay as an in-patient it will inevitably end in a hefty bill. We might take an animal in to give us time to work out what the problem is, or to safeguard its wellbeing, by putting it on a drip for instance, in the interim. It's even worse if the animal ends up having surgery, especially if it's an exploratory laparotomy, when you open up the abdomen just to see what's going on inside. Occasionally an ABC will cost a small fortune, be very lengthy, and produce an end diagnosis of something benign. Good news for the dog, not so good for the owner.

When a case escalates from being simple and straight-forward to being an ABC, you have to explain this to the animal's owner, and this is where things can start to go pear-shaped. People are perfectly ready to accept that their pet may have a complex illness, but not that you can't work out what the illness is, especially when you've had the animal in overnight and done blood tests and X-rays.

Explaining to a client how we try to distinguish a particular disease from others with similar symptoms can be a nightmare. It's a long and tedious business, and for people who aren't used to diagnostic logic it can seem counter-intuitive. But you have to do it, even if some clients don't care: 'Just treat him, I don't want to know.' Often they get stuck on one point and can't get any further. In the end they accept the way we prioritise certain tests and deductions, but they have a problem with the various choices associated with purely medical logic, with the feasibility of tests, and with the cost of the tests; and we do too sometimes, because people are seldom clear about what they want for their pet (apart from the fact that they 'don't want him to suffer').

And then there's the confusion between correlation and its false friend, causality. Just because event A appears to be associated with event B, we shouldn't assume that event A is the cause of event B. Or even that there's any link between them at all.

I once had a spectacular ABC of this kind. A large puppy was brought in on a regular basis by its owners for a string of minor problems. We found a plausible explanation and obtained a satisfactory recovery every time. But the accumulation of mishaps was odd: there were just too many of them.

Then one day the other dog in the household came in from the garden with a bottle that had held a toxic product in its jaws; it showed all the right symptoms, we treated it, and it got better.

For the owners the matter was now cleared up beyond all possible doubt: the puppy had played in that part of the garden on several occasions, and each time it had been poisoned. But for us there was something that didn't fit. For them it was the same thing. And superficially it was. But for us it was impossible, out of the question. Eventually we put our finger on the diagnosis: the puppy had a malformation of the blood vessels in the liver, a rare but classic condition in an unusual and benign presentation. I'm still not sure the owners were convinced.

*

The client in an ABC may be very difficult, thoroughly disagreeable or a complete pain. Or they may be perfectly charming, never let it be said otherwise. In which case the ABC will be far less stressful. Occasionally it is the animal itself that seriously complicates an ABC: spending hours treating a dog that's doing its best to bite you, a feral cat, or an animal that's constantly oozing repulsive and purulent bodily fluids is the very definition of a true vocation.

For an ABC to plumb the depths, the client should ideally make assiduous attempts to help by doing online searches, contacting another vet, or even taking the animal for a second opinion, preferably armed with only some of the test results and none of the details of the diagnostic approach currently being followed.

There's one variation on this last point that reduces me to abject despair. This is when clients start to talk about homeopathy, Bach flower remedies or other forms of 'alternative medicine'. 'Those goddamn bastards have introduced midi-chlorians into the pure sanctity of the Force', or some such claptrap. Just don't bring this nonsense into my work. Or failing that, feel free to carry on without me.

Best of all, though, is when a doctor for humans condescends to meddle in an ABC, tossing a diagnosis or a trenchant comment in my direction, and incidentally putting the animal's life at risk. I dedicate this thought particularly to those endocrinologists and trainee endocrinologists who confuse diabetes in dogs with diabetes in humans.

Sometimes ABCs are known to congregate in gangs. As far as I'm concerned, one ABC in any given week is quite enough. Two or three at a time is sheer hell. That's when I start to lie awake at night.

The ABC is the quintessence of cases that are complex, severe, nuanced, hard to explain, expensive and offer a poor prognosis.

When an ABC works out, I'm a hero. In my own eyes, at least. Sometimes – often, even – the owner remains blissfully unaware. It's no big deal.

When the animal in an ABC dies, I'm sometimes a hero and sometimes an incompetent – and moreover an incompetent who has the brass neck to present the owner with a large bill, to cap it all. Meanwhile I'm in bits, usually.

In the end, an ABC is not that different from an interesting case, just with an extra dose of empathy and emotional investment.

Have you seen my pills?

When I was a vet student, I had an image of organic farmers as youngish, dreadlocked, and with suspicious-looking crops in the woods behind their house. At the same time I viewed them as quite scientific in their approach, choosing organic production methods not only as a reaction against a system that bugged them, but also as a way of fostering certain qualities in their products, not so much in the domain of health and hygiene but more in the area of taste and flavour. I saw them as concerned for the wellbeing of their animals, and stubbornly resistant to any external intervention in their herds.

It's a caricature that doesn't really fit any of the organic farmers whose animals I now treat. Some of them are in their sixties, and none of them sport dreadlocks. In at least a couple of cases I have my suspicions about the crops they grow, but they're not the only ones after all. Some of them are fairly 'scientific', but no more than that. Others are emphatically not, watching their cows grow like dandelions in a field. And not always with poor results, either. Some of them like to ask for lots of advice, often call me, enjoy having a talk, ask me to help with coproscopies before considering worming – that sort of thing. It doesn't give me a lot of work, but then livestock rearing isn't about providing me with a livelihood. 'My' organic farmers may be concerned with the wellbeing of their animals, or not particularly. They may take enormous pride in offering products of the highest quality, or they may care so little that it's depressing.

I also imagined that all organic farmers would be on the left politically, or would vote Green. I never expected to find myself working with an organic farmer who was right-wing. Really, really right-wing. An extremist even. A dyed-in-the-wool supporter of Jean-Marie Le Pen. Maybe of his daughter Marine Le Pen, I don't know. Highly mechanised, highly technical, highly organic, far beyond the required standards currently in force. With a large and splendid herd, moreover, and intelligently farmed land, as far as I can tell. I hardly ever make visits to his farm, as he thinks he knows how to do everything, or at least that I don't know any better than he does. Normally we see each other once a year, for the national prophylactic programme that involves taking a blood sample from every cow and testing it for a range of diseases. I always try to go myself, as I know we'll argue for four or five hours every time.

Well, perhaps not argue exactly, but certainly we'll have a lively discussion. We're never stuck for a topic for debate. Not politics: we did that the first year and kicked it into touch. We avoid the subject now. We focus more on my area, on the medical and hygienic aspects of livestock breeding. It's another field in which he has very definite views. He has his big homeopathy bible, a penchant for Bach flower remedies, and a tendency to believe that if something works once it will work again, every time, and if it doesn't work it's because of something. Or someone.

He's also a great one for conspiracy theories.

And he knows there's nothing I enjoy more than disagreeing with him. I think he likes it too. So we have a discussion. One of us will make some wild generalisation, the other will jump in with both feet, and both of us will argue our point, giving ground only in order to redouble our attacks. As he gets louder and louder, I get quieter and quieter. The cows file past, one by one, and by the time we've exhausted two or three subjects the process will be over. Until the next year.

A few years ago, when I went to vaccinate his cows against malignant catarrhal fever, serious and often fatal, he'd crammed the whole herd into a pen that was too small, intending to send the cows and calves through an exit where I would vaccinate them and take swabs. The pen was really jam-packed, seriously overcrowded. He refused to take some of the herd out to make more space. The worrying thing was that the calves were pushing themselves into the spaces between the cows' legs. Then the inevitable happened: a cow fell down on top of a calf weighing around 100 kilos, fortunately next to the barrier. There was no way we could lift her, as there were other cows more or less falling on top of her. And underneath her, the calf was turning purple. Between three of us we managed to haul it out. It was dead. I intubated it, gave it cardiac massage, injected it with analeptics, and with a good deal of luck managed to resuscitate it. The farmer spent the next couple of hours boasting about the calf that he'd brought back to life by sticking his wretched Bach flower remedies up its snout. Needless to say, my response was scathing.

This year he hit me with something new. He called me out for a cow with a 'uterine infection'. When I got there, I discovered that the cow had given birth a week earlier, that she'd suffered a uterine prolapse (picture the uterus turned inside out like a sock), that he'd put it back in by himself, but only a day later, that the cow had pushed it out again, that he'd pushed it back in again, and hey presto, there we were. I suggested politely that he should call me out for this sort of thing, because when the uterus is put back properly it doesn't come out again, or not usually anyway (it's true it doesn't always work), but he wasn't even listening. 'But the same thing happened a couple of years ago and I put it back no problem!' I explained that there was something else: since the uterus had stayed outside the cow's body for 24 hours it would have had plenty of time to become oedematous, or filled with fluid, for the mucous membranes to become lacerated, and for bacteria to make themselves thoroughly at home. And if he hadn't even disinfected it all before putting it back, it would hardly be surprising if it developed the mother of all infections. And indeed, when I examined the cow I found she was suffering from a raging peritonitis, which might very well prove fatal.

'But I gave her some pills!'

Pills. Homeopathy, you mean. Terrific. Sugar pills
with an 'essence' of something or other that purports to
have some kind of symbolic relationship with the infection or inflammation. Because that's what it's about, isn't
it? Here we have a plant that's supposed to be effective
against inflammation, or else on the contrary it's highly
inflammatory, so according to the theory of 'like cures
like' and that sort of stuff it must be good, so you dilute
it to a maximum of 10 on the 'centesimal scale', meaning that it's diluted by a factor of 100 at each of the ten
stages. In other words, it's like diluting a thimbleful of
alcohol in 100,000,000,000,000,000,000ml of water, or
10,000,000,000,000 cubic metres, or a lake of 100,000
cubic kilometres (for comparison, Lake Geneva contains 89 cubic kilometres of water, though if I'm out by a
couple of zeros please correct me). I have nothing against
plant-based medicines. Plants contain some highly active
molecules. But I draw the line at homeopathy. I don't
doubt that homeopathy can obtain excellent results among
human patients, notably through the placebo effect (and
here I'm being completely serious), and that many illnesses
get better by themselves if you wait a bit, even sometimes
in veterinary medicine. But there are limits.

So. Personally, my thing is more evidence-based medicine. Science, real science, is perpetually self-questioning;
it checks and rechecks its results, dismisses anything that
doesn't work (even if people have believed in it for ever),
and constantly re-examines its premises.

And besides, there's no logic whatever in the way he uses homeopathy. He's got a big book on the subject, and he falls back on two or three 'recipes' – ready-made and bought over the counter – that have 'worked' once, and that he now uses like magic spells.

What I'm happy about on this occasion is that he gives me a hearing. And his son even more so: given the sort of man his father is, it can't be often that he sees anyone stand up to him.

What I'm less happy about is that despite the uterine flush, anti-inflammatories and antibiotics I've given her, the cow's chances of pulling through are slim. The peritonitis will probably gradually gain a hold, and she'll fade away and die.

I just hope he doesn't come out with some remark along the lines of 'your antibiotics didn't work any better than my pills'. If he does, though, I'm one step ahead of him. I told him that the treatment started too late. That she should have had the antibiotics when the prolapse happened, not when her intestines were flooded with fibrin. That her chances of survival were vanishingly small. He heard me out, but ...

We'll see soon enough.

Donkeys

'Doctor, our donkey's just had a baby foal!'
'Oh?'

'Yes, it's her third foal. A female!'

'Oh?'

'...'

'Is the mother OK? Is there something wrong with the foal?'

'No, no, nothing wrong. It's just that it's the third in three years!'

'Mmm, or a bit longer I'd have thought, given the gestation period of a donkey. Is she with the male?'

'Yes, yes, we've got a pair, but tell me, do female donkeys have a foal every year all their lives?'

'Mmm, pretty much.'

'But that's terrible! What are we going to do with all those donkeys? I mean, this is the third one after all!'

'All females?'

'Yes, they're lovely.'

'And soon they'll be mothers ...'

'Oh no, they're with their father, you see.'

'…'

'Are you still there?'

'Yes, er, well that doesn't mean he won't cover them.'

'It doesn't?'

'Well, if …'

'But … so what should we do?'

'The simplest thing in your case, Madame, would be to geld the father.'

'Oh! We couldn't do that! Poor thing!'

'Or else buy another field.'

'Ahh. Um, to have him gelded, would it cost a lot?'

'Less than a field …'

To treat them
is to love them

At vet school, we learned all about empathy and its false friend, sympathy. We were trained to anticipate mental blocks and to avoid them, and we were helped to understand not only the bonds of attachment between pets and their owners, but also the way in which money matters and medical matters are inextricably intertwined in our profession. We were taught to explain, to communicate, to enhance our work. We were shown the importance of both style and substance. We were prepared for the delicate business of imparting news, especially bad news – good news is easy. We were given advice on how to deal with putting an animal down. In short, we were taught all about the human side of our future profession, in the broadest sense of the term.

I'm joking, of course. In fact we weren't taught a single thing about any of this. Absolutely nothing at all. Instead we had to learn off endless lists of symptoms and diseases, medicines and parasites: everything that you'd imagine, basically, as well as quite a lot that you wouldn't imagine, such as statistics, electrostatics and thermodynamics. I liked thermodynamics.

But no one told us whether or not we were supposed to like our clients, the owners of our patients, the farmers, the horse riders and all the rest. And I have to say the question never even occurred to me.

It should have gone without saying that, yes, of course we'd like our patients. After all, everyone knows you want to be a vet because-you-like-animals. But this was an area in which the coldly clinical nature of our teaching was about to make us question ourselves.

When I started out as a vet, I was the product of my education and training, like everyone else. I was opposed to hunting and bullfighting, racism and homophobia. I was in favour of world peace. And of having a sense of humour. I was opposed to religion, but I was in favour of positive Christian values – I'd been to Sunday school, after all. I wasn't a vegetarian, and I'm still not. I was for, or I was against. Animals had to be treated, but not at any price: there was a limit, of course there was, I just never wanted to come up against it. I nurtured the idea that I would be discerning and nuanced in my approach.

Now nothing is so clear any more. Not that I'm in favour of hunting and bullfighting, or racism and homophobia, any more than I'm against world peace. But now I find I can like people who go hunting, as well as total cretins of racist conspiracy theorists. I can like eco-minded people of the far right as well as of the far left. I can like owners who are violent, who mistreat their animals, who neglect them, who are pig-ignorant. I can like men and women of every description. I don't necessarily enjoy their company. I think I understand them quite often. I rarely agree with them, or rather I do, but only on some things. And I don't have that many friends. I'm a long way from where I grew up, and I've been assiduous in not making friends. Not always successfully, I'm happy to say. Even if treating animals that belong to people I've grown close to can be complicated.

There are lots of my clients who I don't find particularly appealing. Often they're everything I'm not, everything I could never be.

But I'm fond of them.

I'm fond of the right-wing organic farmer. I'm attached to his twisted logic and his stubborn certainties.

I'm fond of the great beanpole of a half-witted teenager who quite simply let his dog die.

I'm fond of the couple with slight learning difficulties who adopted a new kitten the day their old cat died. The new kitten was called Tigrée, the old cat was Noireaude.

Noireaude was huge. Shut up in their tiny apartment with Monsieur who chain-smoked like an A&E doctor, Noireaude used to cough and throw up. They doted on her.

The first time I met them, they had an emergency appointment because Monsieur had punished Noireaude as a kitten – for I don't know what trifling offence – by crashing her head against the sink. She had a minor traumatic brain injury. It was a distressing incident, and I had to explain to them very simply and clearly how to tell a kitten off. By holding it by the scruff of the neck and saying 'no', firmly but calmly. The level of their handicap wasn't so severe that I could let them off completely and unreservedly, but they just needed to have it explained to them. And in any case, how had they themselves been punished in their time?

They didn't have children. They had Noireaude instead. Noireaude who was bored. Noireaude who was restless, who miaowed, who was always clamouring for attention. The only way they could calm her down was by feeding her. And so she got fatter and fatter; she'd wolf down her food, then throw it up again. And then she'd stop eating altogether for a couple of days.

So they'd bring her in to see me, and every time I'd search in vain for anything wrong. It became a bit of a joke. And they'd always insist on seeing me. They wanted to try everything. So did we. High-fibre diet food. Stuff to help fur balls pass through. Because yes, she'd also pull out clumps of fur, swallow them and then bring them up again.

Noireaude was going crazy.

We told them this, in every possible way. We tried to find some way for her to be able to go outside, we tried to negotiate toys for her, space, freedom. They wouldn't have any of it. They were too frightened that she'd be run over. They'd take her out now and then on a leash and harness. Just what she needed to put the cap on her frustration.

We tried anxiolytic pheromones to reduce her anxiety levels. With a bit of success, but not enough. We decided against giving her a stronger dose, as pills would never be the complete answer. Would we have to knock her out? Every time Noireaude started yowling again, Madame would pop an anti-anxiety pill. And in the morning she'd come to see me.

'I haven't slept a wink all night.'

And I could never find anything wrong, nothing at all.

Until the day when I did find something. You had to stay on the alert, and not just heave a sigh and go through the motions. You had to be aware that this time there was something different. That there was something behind all this vomiting.

Noireaude had lost weight. And not because of the diet.

Noireaude had stopped yowling. And not because of the pheromones.

So I put Noireaude down. I'd spent an hour explaining the complications and nuances of her illness to her owners, and they agreed straight away. Madame took her pills. Monsieur went outside for a cigarette.

And later that same day they came back with Tigrée.

But this time I was ready for them. I was going to become a dispenser of justice, sort of. I'd have to exaggerate a bit perhaps, to lie to them possibly, to be manipulative certainly. But Tigrée would be allowed to go outside, Tigrée would have her freedom. Tigrée would be able to escape from the gloom, the fug and the pills. She'd be able to get away from her owners who didn't know how to love her.

You can always hope.

A world of pain

Just a normal Sunday on call. It's half past eleven, the morning's nearly over, and things seem to be calming down at last. I'm so tired – not quite on automatic pilot, just exhausted. I'm praying that the afternoon will be uneventful.

One last tour of the kennels, a check on all the drips, and I'm off.

Except that's the phone again. We have a friend staying, and I've got a feeling I won't be having lunch with him and the family.

Hold that smile.

'Hello, out-of-hours service.'

'Oh hello, I'm calling about Nestor, his back legs are paralysed, he can't get up, he has to drag himself on his front legs when he needs to go out.'

OK, this is the emergency call no one wants. The dog's probably been paralysed for a while, his life isn't in danger, but he'll be in unbearable pain. A herniated disc, acute arthritis or something else, I don't want to put it off till later and spend the whole of lunch thinking about it. So let's get on with it.

'Can you bring him in straight away?'

'OK, straight away, my son will bring him, thanks a lot!'

'And what about y—'

He's gone. No time to ask who he is, where he's coming from, how long it will take to get here. I text home to tell them not to wait for me, and I get on with drawing up the weekly order for drugs and other supplies.

When that's done, I chase up late payments. Flick through a few articles. It's a quarter past twelve. It's over half an hour now that I've been waiting for this guy. I bet he's not going to turn up. I'll give him till half past, then I'm off.

It's 25 past when he arrives. Of course. As I go out to his car with him, I enquire politely what took him so long. He explains that he couldn't find the car keys.

There on the back seat is Nestor. A twelve-year-old German shepherd. He looks at me uncertainly and makes a vague attempt to wag his tail. He exudes pain, he's the embodiment of suffering. His features are emaciated, his back legs have wasted away, his undercoat is sticking out in grimy tufts, and he reeks of urine. His back paws are tensed and pointing forwards and his back is arched, braced on his front paws. He pants at me and says hello, just like all the other dogs that keep on wagging their tails however much misery we inflict on them.

I have no wish to talk to his owner. I was cross already because he was late, but I'm grown-up enough not to mention it. Probably he genuinely had lost his keys, which is stupid but not serious. And then there's something about this great awkward stammering lump, barely out of his teens, standing there like a wilting maize stalk, with his spectacles and his too-tight jumper, his Citroën AX and his loafers, that makes me want to hug him even more than I want to hit him. But the fact remains that a whole history of chronic suffering is bound up in this heap of matted fur on the back seat of the car, this great rock of canine devotion. Of unconditional love.

It makes me want to cry.

I don't even speak to the tall, dark-haired youth; instead I carry the dog into the surgery, holding him under the chest, his back legs dangling. He barely emits a whimper and tries to give me an awkward going over with his tongue. I put him down in a heap on the table in the consulting room and give him a rapid clinical examination.

He's thin, but not exaggeratedly so. His hindquarters are bony and stiff, the muscles little more than tendons. The silence is making the youth uncomfortable, so he tries a couple of opening gambits. Talking to him is the last thing I want to do, but I need to know.

'How long has he been like this?'

'A couple of days.'

'And you didn't call me before?'

I'm not angry, I'm not angry, I'm not angry.

'Well, erm, it's my brother's dog, he's back tomorrow, but I thought it couldn't wait because he had to crawl outside to do his business. He hasn't done a poo since the day before yesterday.'

Imbecile!

'OK, has he peed at least?'

'Yes, on the grass, he dragged himself out and did it half sitting down, with his back legs stuck out.'

Don't raise your voice. It won't do any good. It won't help the dog.

'Fine, we're going to do an X-ray, I think he's got a major problem with his back. Is that OK with you?'

Yes. It is. Of course it is.

'Er, OK, if you think so.'

'Was he stiff before this?'

Of course he was stiff before this.

'Yeah, he was.'

'For how long?'

'Maybe two or three years?'

'Two or three *years*?'

Did you hear it, the menace in my voice?

'How stiff?'

'Well, he's had trouble getting up in the morning.'

'He's been dragging his back legs when he walks, he's had difficulty getting up stairs and into the car?'

'Yeah, that's right.'

'For two or three years?'

'Yeah, at least that.'

'Has he been on any medication?'

Say yes.

'Um, no.'

'Fine. We'll do that X-ray then.'

I give the dog an injection of anti-inflammatories and another of a morphine-type drug.

'What are they for?'

'For the pain. He's in pain.'

'Oh, OK.'

I don't feel like shouting any more. I feel like weeping. I want to be hard and unpleasant, but I just feel like dissolving in tears. To be absolutely clear, when I called him a 'great awkward stammering lump' I wasn't being entirely fair. This young man isn't a complete idiot, far from it. He doesn't have the excuse of suffering from learning difficulties. He's just a normal bloke. Someone like you or me. Someone you might pass in the street.

I pick the dog up in my arms and carry him to the radiology room. I switch the developing machine on, position the plate and put on the lead-lined apron, thyroid shield and protective goggles.

'Woah, it's like a suit of armour!'

'Yes, to protect against X-rays. Leave the room, please.'

What was that smart-arse remark about? Is he taking the piss or what? Doesn't he realise that his dog is probably going to die? That I'll almost certainly have to put him down? Do I look as if I'm in a mood for jokes? It's not as if I'm being exactly friendly or even polite, except when I address him with a professional courtesy that gets me out of having to talk to him more directly.

I put the old dog on his side, make the necessary adjustments. When I speak gently to him, he wags his tail. Feebly, timidly, with all the enthusiasm that his pain allows. In the silence I stroke him gently. He doesn't dare turn his head, and he watches me out of the corner of his eye with a look of frustrated love, the look of a dog who wants to leap into my arms but quite simply can't.

I call his owner back in. He needs to be with the dog while I go to develop the X-rays, to make sure he doesn't hurt himself by trying to do anything acrobatic like clamber down from the table.

When I return to the radiology room, the only sounds as I wait for the X-ray to develop are the hum of the developing machine and the mewing of a cat that I operated on during the night. Neither of us says a word, and the great lump sways from side to side, looking ill at ease. He can't bear a silence.

'Euuggh, must be horrendous being on call all day with those cats on heat screeching for a tom.'

'I operated on that cat last night. I removed her uterus, ovaries and three decomposing kittens. She's not on heat, she's all alone, lost and in pain.'

That should shut him up. No?

'But still, moggies on heat, a total nightmare, huh? Tee hee.'

Finally the wretched X-ray is developed, which means I don't have to find an answer. I glance at it against the infrared lamp. Just as I thought. I'll show him a normal X-ray first.

'So. This is a normal dog's spine. Here are the vertebrae, the pelvis, the ribs and the stomach. You can clearly see the rounded edges of the vertebrae and the processes, these bony projections. So this is all good. Now, this is Nestor.'

On hearing his name, Nestor wags his tail. Or tries to.

'Nestor's spine is non-existent. Over the past two or three years, he's developed crippling arthritis. The bone spurs have fused, the sacrum has fused with the lumbar vertebrae, the lumbar vertebrae have fused with the thoracic vertebrae, he has zero mobility left in his spine, he's got a pickaxe handle where he should have a spinal column. He's been in pain for two or three years, and he's been suffering in silence. Then a couple of days ago he suffered a severe herniated disc. He'd probably had minor ones before, but this one caused a compression of the spinal cord that's so serious that the nerve impulses can no longer travel along it, and Nestor can't move his back legs. He's paralysed. Either because of the pain, or because of the compression of the nerves, or both. I'm pretty sure it's the compression though.'

I say it quickly. Firmly. Clearly. I look him straight in the eye. His eyes are brimming, and great tears are rolling down his cheeks. He's snivelling, breaking down, this overgrown kid who I want to beat to death with spinal bone spurs, who I want to comfort and hug tight. He blows his nose noisily, sniffs and splutters.

'But what can you *dooooooo*?' he wails.

'He's your brother's dog?'

'Yeah ...'

'I suggest I keep him in till tonight. That will give time for the morphine and anti-inflammatories to take effect. If he can stand up tonight, then it's the pain, and we can try to manage it. If not, there's no point in kidding ourselves.

Surgery can't help, and this is no life for him. We'll have to put him down.'

Ten minutes later, Nestor is in his cage. It's two o'clock and I'm starving; there were flashes in front of my eyes as I explained the X-ray to the lad. I wait for him to drive out of the car park before I leave. I have no desire to encounter him again. While I wait, I put all the orders and bills to one side, and I make a fuss of Nestor, cradling his great brave German shepherd head in my hand as he enjoys the feel of my fingers ruffling his fur, the sound of my whispered words of comfort.

When I leave the surgery the kid's still there, sitting in the driving seat of his car with the door open and legs outside, holding his head in his hands. I stop to see if he's OK.

'I've broken *dooooooown*!' He's wailing again. 'I've got a flat battery, I haven't got a mobile, I live twenty kilometres away!'

You don't say.

I get the jump leads (you can find anything at this surgery), put my vehicle bonnet to bonnet with his, and get it started. I watch him as he sets off, just to be sure he doesn't plough the car into one of the plane trees that line the road.

I loathe him, and I love him. I'm quite sure I was once as dumb as he is. By tonight his dog will be dead. I just hope that the dog's owner will have grown up a bit.

*

There wasn't a miracle.

When I went back to see him at seven o'clock that evening, Nestor was waiting for me in his cage. Sitting up. I got him out of the cage, and tried to help him walk a few steps. It was no use. The nerves were destroyed and he had a herniated disc with major compression, there was no doubt about it. I put Nestor back in his cage. He was wagging his tail furiously, with all the enthusiasm of a dog that was no longer in pain, of a dog who'd discovered that the world could be a different place, goddammit.

I called his owner to tell him. His brother and father confirmed that they wanted him put down.

So I went back to the kennels, where Nestor's tail was still drumming out an ode to unconditional joy. I stroked him, I inserted a catheter, talking to him all the while, whispering a stream of foolish nothings that filled him with delight. All that dumb canine devotion. I got out a tin of cat food, the luxury stuff. He started devouring it, delirious with joy. It was as he pushed his muzzle deep into the tin that I injected him, that he collapsed.

IIe fell asleep, his tail wagging ever more feebly, his jowls festooned with flecks of cat food.

I talked to him, but he couldn't hear me any more. No more suffering. No more happiness. No more pain. No more wild enthusiasm. No more love.

I euthanised him, and I listened as his heart stopped beating, until the last fibrillation.

Then I took a big white bag and I put him into it.

Pirouette

Listen.
A heart beating.
A litany, a simple sound.
Listen.
So as not to see, so as not to hear.
So as not to be aware of their tears.
Big kids, old people.
Terrified, or agonised.
Impotent.
Listen.
A heart beating.
My stethoscope, eyes closed.
Listen.
Don't cry, don't go under.
Run away, run or hide.
Far away from these people, from the here and now.
Cared for, fussed over.
He's going ...
A heartbeat missed.
The rhythm's going, the tempo weeps

Of rebellion, one last clarion call.

Fibrillation.

The sound fades slowly. The blood ebbs away.

Now there's nothing

But this heart, this rhythm, this beat, this pulse.

I am gone, he has left me,

I am sitting close beside him.

They are here

But this lonely heart

Beats only for me now

Only I hear its music.

Only I hear the coma.

For a few minutes, a few beats,

I gather up this last breath,

This fugue.

Softly.

Silently.

The final witness.

Without pain, without suffering,

Far away from all these people, all these children, all these teenagers and their parents.

His last pirouette

Was for them.

His last heartbeat

Was for me.

'He's gone.

It's over.'

Kids of all ages

It's just on eleven o'clock in the morning as I remove my arm from the cow's birth canal.

'Uterine torsion, 270 degrees, irreducible, nothing to be done. We'll have to open her up.'

In the minutes that follow, old men, neighbours and other curious onlookers roll up to enjoy the major spectacle of a caesarean. The setting is perfect, with a clear, transparent light, clean straw and a gentle breeze. The cattle are lowing, the birds are singing, the smell of the cows mingles with the aroma of damp grass drying in the September sunshine. Cleaning, disinfection, incision: I ask the latest old codger to arrive to pass me the metal box containing my surgical instruments.

'Without touching anything inside it, please.'

He's stuck his great fingers inside the box, but – caught in the nick of time – he doesn't touch anything. Hmmm, OK then. Tall, stiff, his face bronzed by the sun under his cap, brown trousers and shirt of an indefinable blue, he starts mucking about with the farmer who's standing beside me, leaning his weight against the heifer.

When I next turn round, the 85-year-old is miming making a surgical incision in the farmer's stomach, a little smile on his face, his eyes creased with wrinkles of happiness.

Sweet.

The scrape of metal. I turn round quickly. The old boy's still pretending to cut the farmer open, but this time with my scalpel in his right hand.

I explode.

'What the hell do you think you're playing at?'

He protests in disbelief:

'But I wasn't really going to do it!'

He's trying to justify himself. Now I don't believe it.

'I don't give a damn if you cut him open!'

I'm speaking very clearly.

'But ...'

He's like a child.

'Listen, my instruments are sterile, and your hands are filthy. Are you crazy or what? That goes in the cow's stomach, goddammit!'

In a flash he puts the scalpel back in the box. Just like that. Genius. That's all sorted then.

After that he doesn't say a word, doesn't move a muscle except to anticipate my movements when I turn round to get a needle or a clamp.

Kids! Octogenarian kids!

The calf in the hearth

It was one of those freezing cold late afternoons in April. A Sunday, typically. A long way from home, a long way from the comfort of my living room, a long way from the central heating. A long way from springtime.

That morning you could almost have believed that spring was in the air. Then came the drizzle, fine, penetrating and persistent, to shatter the illusion.

'He was born this morning, I saw his mother was licking him, so I came back to the house. When I went back at about five, he wasn't moving. I brought him back here in the tractor bucket.'

The calf is stretched out, his head thrown backwards and his eyes rolled back. He's shaking. No pupil reflex, heart OK. Not yet twelve hours old and already suffering from hypothermia. My thermometer registers his temperature at 33.5 degrees.

He hasn't moved.

'He's dying of cold, your calf.'

A bit like me, but worse. Now that's what you call diagnostic skill.

'I'm going to need a bucket of hot water, really hot, hot water bottles, containers of scalding water and straw, to start with.'

He's not dehydrated, but his blood pressure must be low. Everything must be low. A saline drip with sugar. I add corticoids and an antibiotic to the bottle as a precaution. A little vitamin E, just because, and an intravenous hypertonic saline solution administered rapidly as a bolus dose. Belt and braces.

The guy comes back with a bucket of water. I plunge the bottle into it along with the line to two IV solution bags, so that the liquid can stay in the hot water as long as possible before reaching the calf's jugular. The farmer watches me with the look of a newborn calf when it sees a cat for the first time: curious, fascinated even, but utterly dazed. As he would later tell me, he'd never heard of an intravenous sugar solution. And all my endless lines, all screwed into each other! A veterinary take on make-do-and-mend, and one of the great charms of the profession. Thinking on your feet, falling back on your own nous and resources, cobbling together DIY contraptions, whatever it takes to save a life!

He's also brought me two bottles of scalding water. Of course, as if three litres of water will be enough to warm up a 50-kilo calf. I don't say anything, just position them against the infant. I have twenty minutes to kill in any case, the time the sodding drip will take. Nice and slow. If I can just get the needle into the wretched jugular of a calf suffering from low blood pressure! Which doesn't show any reaction, more to the point.

Twenty minutes during which I can explain to the farmer that by a hot water bottle I mean at least 40 litres. He must have some containers lying about somewhere, surely? That the drugs and drips are all very well, but what the calf really needs is to warm up. That his mother can't have licked him for very long, that he's been left soaking wet in the freezing rain and mud, that he probably hasn't suckled, that he might have a slightly underactive thyroid, which is common hereabouts. If he survives, we'll give him some iodine and selenium. Yes, yes, lots of vitamins will be a good thing, but it's not vitamins that will save him, Monsieur ...

Twenty minutes later, I struggle to stand up again, my legs seized after kneeling down for so long. The drip's done, the calf is still dying, still frozen.

The farmer, meanwhile, continues to watch me, wringing his hands. Evidently the message about the hot water bottles hasn't got through. Too delicately phrased, doubtless. So I get to the point.

'It would be good to get him inside, too. Could we get him in the garage, beside the boiler? Or is there a fire lit in the house?'

He watches me, eyes wide with terror, as I go back to the car to write out the pointless prescription spelling out the waiting time needed before the meat can be consumed from a calf that will die tonight.

He stands there waiting.

'Have you got a fire lit?'

'Oh, yes, would you like a coffee?'

OK. I'm strong, and I'm a vet.

I lift the calf up in my arms. He dangles like a corpse, but a corpse that's breathing. He's a dead weight.

The farmer rolls his eyes.

As I head for the house, he trots along beside me. The calf weighs as much as a donkey, but I'm a vet, I'm a man, I'm strong, I smile casually, I hold my breath. It's bloody miles back to the house! It must be at least ten kilometres! And the house must be at least 500 metres higher than the cowshed!

A couple of minutes later, the farmer opens the blasted door to the blasted house and slips inside in front of me, with an air of he-who-obeys. Another door. A proper airlock before the inner sanctum, the living room with its great brick fireplace, as big as an inglenook almost. Sweeping the poker out of the way with my muddy boot, I deposit the calf on the hearth.

There's a dead body on Madame's hearth. The dead body of a calf. But it's breathing!

'So it's going to die then?'

'More than likely, Madame, and if he survives there will no doubt be after-effects, but if he stays outside he'll certainly die. He's suffering from hypothermia, he has to warm up, it's too cold in the cowshed.'

By now Monsieur has virtually disappeared under the table. A magnificent, immaculately polished oak table, on a superb and flawlessly clean tiled floor. An impeccably ironed table runner. Gleaming copper ornaments. Not a speck of dust on the fireplace. Little slippers in the re-entry. The trail left by my muddy boots. The dead body of a calf breathing on the hearth. It's that breathing that I cling on to.

It would have been better to do the drip here, in the warm.

Neither of them dares breathe a word. I brazenly exploit my vet's aura to claim this space for the newborn. Here, in this world that's about 200 kilometres away from the cowshed. At least.

And I slip away.

The calf did pull through in the end. The farmer still talks about it. I haven't seen his wife since. The calf spent a night in the warm. Their niece visited them that evening, a few hours after I'd left. She suggested taking some photos of the calf in the hearth, but he wouldn't have it: he didn't want any souvenirs of that dead calf in his house.

He regrets it now. The calf survived and is in rude health, without any ill effects. Not one.

My sodium chloride and dextrose drip with two lines is now famous locally. I'd also added a vitamin solution that was coloured red, so red is now absolutely the last word.

There are times when you perform truly virtuoso feats of diagnosis or surgery, and there isn't a soul there to appreciate them.

And there are others when you cobble something together with two bits of plastic and you do something inconceivable. Like carrying a calf inside a house. And it's the talk of the town.

Go figure.

Brave

I remember the panic in her voice, the darkness of the bedroom, the still of the night shattered by the ringing of the on-call mobile.

I remember her words, the visceral fear and razor-sharp clarity with which she'd grasped the distinction between a benign incident and the death of a companion. You didn't need to be a vet, that night, to realise that this was an absolute emergency.

'He's shaking, he was sleeping peacefully, his breathing is terribly laboured and he's making a dreadful noise!'

I remember my sense of resignation, as soon as I realised that I was 30 kilometres from Brave, with the surgery halfway in between. I told her to put her dog in the car and meet me there.

'But will he be able to cope with the journey? Couldn't you come to us?'

'Time is of the essence, we need oxygen, and we need the equipment at the surgery.'

'But what if he dies on the way there?'

'If it's that much of an emergency, I wouldn't be able to do anything for him anyway.'

Cold logic, born of experience and empiricism. She understood completely. There was no time left, not a minute to spare.

I remember the second call on the mobile, two minutes later, as I was pulling on my jacket and heading out to the vehicle, knowing all the while that there was no point. I knew she was calling to tell me that Brave was dead.

I remember the tears in her voice, the lamentation.

I remember the desperate loneliness, the violence of her grief.

Brave was dead, and there was nothing more I could say. But what was my impotence in the face of her grief?

I stammered out a few words that wouldn't reach her now, not yet, but that might perhaps help her later not to blame herself. If I could at least give her that?

The call can't have lasted even as much as a minute. There was nothing to be said. Just tears and silence. Grief and impotence.

I remember the blood drained from my face.

All these years I've remembered Brave and his young mistress, the fiancé who'd bought him for her and who had left him with her when he moved out, the accidents and minor mishaps, the worries and joys, Brave as a puppy and Brave as an old dog. I've remembered a dog's life, and a piece of a human life.

Colic

Alouette is waiting.

Sheltered from the wind, in the passage between the loose boxes and the hay bales, the bay mare is more comfortable now, after the medication I've given her for her attacks of colic. She could die. From shock, or from pain.

In the rickety stable silence reigns, despite the deafening howling of the wind between the corrugated iron sheets of the roof. There are five of us. Madame Tolzac, two of her friends, my work experience student and me. We're all looking at the young woman, and over her shoulder at the old mare waiting patiently, relieved after the removal of her nasogastric tube. Between Madame Tolzac and me is the bucket containing the reflux siphoned off by the nasogastric tube: ten litres of water, paraffin oil and unidentifiable stuff that would be more at home in the mare's intestines or stomach, where I had sent them a few hours earlier, on my first visit.

Intestinal transit has seized up again, although the anti-inflammatories will still be working. It was only a quarter of an hour ago, moreover, that I allowed myself a huge smile of relief when a belly tap, puncturing the abdominal wall, had revealed the absence of peritonitis and gastrointestinal rupture. But this bucket of reflux is seriously bad news, casting a gloomy shadow over any optimism we might have felt. The illness is still out of control. The mare is still distended by intestinal gases, even if she doesn't appear to be in too much pain.

I have to make some phone calls. I've managed the emergency and I've reached my limits. Of course there's more I can do. A caecal tap, abdominal decompression, a drip, drugs containing morphine. But the longer I wait, the slimmer the mare's chances if I get it wrong. Or if she needs surgery.

*

'We should be able to find a specialist vet in this area who can take her. They'll be able to give a better diagnosis and provide you with a prognosis. Suggest surgery, if necessary. Medically, there are a few more things I can do, pretty much everything we *can* do in cases of colic. But it might not be enough, and I don't have many diagnostic tools. You need to decide now, as Alouette's condition could worsen and it might be too late. So I suggest we call a specialist colleague to ask their advice.'

She says:

'How much would that cost?'

She's still shivering. From the cold?

'I don't know, I'll ask. A consultation and hospitalisation would be reasonable, for sure. Surgery would be much less reasonable though. Fifteen hundred euros, at least. I don't know.'

She drops the cigarette she's in the middle of rolling. I'm on my mobile before she can say a word.

I manage to get through to the first colleague I call. He's snowed under, with three cases of colic in his clinic already. He can't see her, but he gives me some rapid words of advice instead. He's not reassuring. A second call, I go through it all again:

'A mare, seventeen years old, on heat, high levels of small strongyle worms, partial response to anti-spasmodics given by her owner and anti-inflammatories added by me. Moderate tachycardia, no fever, but she's been struggling for a while: could it be parasites? Or piroplasmosis? We're waiting for the results of tests. Her abdomen is distended, her owner says. Palpation reveals a mass of intestines with a build-up of gas, with no change since this morning. Six hours ago I did an NGI without any problem, no reflux, paraffin, magnesium sulphate, bicarbonates. This evening ten litres of reflux, containing all I administered to her this morning. Paracentesis normal. Could you take her in? And if she needs surgery what would the estimated cost be?'

No time for my colleague to get a word in edgeways. He asks for a couple of details, and then, very quietly, he gives me his answer. He can take her in no problem, but if he has to operate the starting price would be 3,000 euros.

I thank him and hang up, saying I'll call back in a few minutes. Then I issue Madame Tolzac with an ultimatum. I tell her she has to make a decision now, on the spot. Does she

want to take Alouette to my colleague or not? If the treatment I've given turns out to be successful, it could all be for
nothing. On the other hand, she'd get a better diagnosis, a
prognosis, possibly a more specific medical treatment, and
in the worst-case scenario the option of surgery.

*

Madame Tolzac tries to light her cigarette again, nearly
drops it again, apologises for smoking near the hay, struggles to speak, chokes, tries not to cry. She's spent the last
three minutes rolling that cigarette, the automatic, habitual movements failing to conceal the shaking of her hands.
Alouette's tether rests on her shoulder.

She heaves a sigh, takes a deep breath, abandons her
roll-up. She's stopped shaking, but she looks as if she's on
the verge of tears. She hesitates. Standing there, in the middle of her tumbledown stable with its salvaged corrugated
metal roof, its improvised loose boxes and its hay bales,
surrounded by her rescue horses – animals that have been
put out to grass, abandoned because they were too old
or mistreated – she gives me her answer, half-swallowing
her words:

'I haven't got money like that. And if I could find it and
I spent it on Alouette, then the others would have nothing
to eat, and I wouldn't be able to make this place work at
all. So there's no point in going to see the specialist if he
can't really do anything more without surgery. We'll have
to do what we can here, we'll have to make do with what
we've got.'

So over the next three days, I punctured, drained, cath-
eterised, transfused, administered morphine, gave advice,
wormed, and answered all her calls. I thought of all the
horses I'd seen throwing themselves against the walls of
their stables in pain. I thought about the ones that had
collapsed. About the ones I'd had to put down because I
couldn't save them.

There were some highs over those three days, quite a
few of them, and some lows. Alouette pulled out her drip,
the catheter got folded back. She escaped to be with her
foal. There was no rapid improvement, and it was a while
before we dared to hope for the best. I went back to see
her again, twice.

*

Alouette did pull through.

*

In this strange unequal lottery, this weighted contest in
which the means existed but were beyond our reach, we
took a punt. We gambled, and this time we won.

Mad cow?

He called me because his cow was behaving bizarrely. And the way he told me about it was odd, too. He sounded a bit embarrassed. I'd assumed he was afraid it was BSE, mad cow disease, the worst thing that can happen to a cattle farmer. I wasn't unduly concerned: we've got rid of BSE.

He was calling about a Holstein, a black-and-white dairy cow. She was five or six years old, nice and plump, had just calved after a good match.

All hunky-dory.

'She's gone crazy. She's all skittish, like a kid goat, she's licking the walls, and she's giving me such weird looks!'

Ah.

And on top of all that, her breath smelt nicely of acetone. Ketosis is a classic condition in dairy cattle, the result of an accumulation of ketones following the massive mobilisation of fats in the early stages of lactation. It occurs quite frequently in cows that are too fat when they calve, and that produce a lot of milk. The ketones, with their distinctive smell of pear drops, spread throughout the cow's body and cause nervous disorders, generally benign and completely reversible. The cows go a little crazy, but not mad as in BSE. It's easily diagnosed by the pear-drop smell and confirmed with a straightforward urine test strip, and the treatment is simple and aimed at putting the cow's metabolism back on an even keel.

As I was chatting to the farmer and preparing the drips and injections, the Holstein was standing just behind us. Without warning, she suddenly lunged at him, her mouth wide open. As I jumped out of the way and landed in a heap in the straw, the cow clamped her jaws round the farmer's belt and yanked his trousers down around his ankles. Then she let go and resumed her place.

'That's the fourth time she's done that this morning!'

And she did it one more time while we were doing her transfusions.

No doubt about it, she was in love.

All hunky-dory? The jury's out.

The first time

It was somewhere in the region of Nantes. I was 23. I wasn't yet a doctor of veterinary surgery, and I'd only just qualified as a veterinary physician. I was doing an internship in a large and almost exclusively rural practice, with a density of livestock that was truly mind-boggling. That still is, doubtless. The vets in that practice were responsible for 50,000 head of cattle a year, meaning they were treating 50,000 adult cows, each of which calved every year. Virtually all of them Charolais.

The team would carry out four or five caesareans every night. I say 'the team', as a single out-of-hours vet wouldn't have been able to cope. They worked in pairs, at least, with another pair as back-up. And I went with them, day and night. I was on a steep learning curve, calving a breed with which no one ever takes any risks, so high are the chances that the calf will get stuck on the way out.

I also learned how to calve a cow the traditional way, with all the subtleties of manipulating the calf *in utero*, and everything you need to know and do. In this practice, though, these were risks that weren't often taken, and for good reason: in this practice, they operated. Charolais cattle are an excellent learning tool for surgery, not so much for obstetrics.

The clinic also treated dogs and cats. The younger vets there had realised that there was a demand for it, that it wasn't enough any more to just give a dog an injection when you happened to be visiting the farm. They had invested in training and equipment. And in time. The older vets weren't keen, but they could see the relevance of this newfangled development and they put up with it.

On this particular day, it was the senior vet of the practice who was conducting a surgery for dogs. Dr Vailleux was an old-school vet in the textbook mould: his shirts and trousers were always crisply laundered and ironed, he lived in a substantial family house, and he drove a top-of-the-range car that he kept scrupulously, gleamingly clean. 'It doesn't take any longer to be clean and tidy in your work', was his axiom, the principle that he did his best to drill into me, whether the matter in hand was surgical methods, cars or boots. With varying degrees of success, to judge by the state of my car. 'It's not just a matter of the quality of your work, but also of the image you project.' The leather seats in his car didn't even smell of cows.

He had known the time when every village had its vet, or couple of vets. Now vets formed group practices, and had bought up any vets who held out in single practice. He was a pillar of local society, in a way that his younger colleagues would never be.

That day, Dr Vailleux was seeing an elderly couple. He

knew them well, as they'd had cattle. He let me examine their bitch, an elderly, worn-out German shepherd cross.

I didn't say much to them, listening instead to their answers to the scant questions he asked them. The diagnosis was obvious, even to me. A purulent vaginal discharge: I did a scan, which confirmed pyometra, a uterine infection. The next step was equally simple: check for absence of kidney failure and operate. There was no real alternative.

I don't think Dr Vailleux even explained the diagnosis to the old couple. I can't remember exactly how he phrased it, but basically he told them she was done for. They stood up, shook his hand, thanked him respectfully and left, all the while doing their best to hide their feelings. Dr Vailleux left the dog to me.

'Right then, you can put her down.'

I stood there, rooted to the spot.

Not rooted to the spot as in *but I'm here to treat her*; as in, 'But that's monstrous, there's no question of my killing a dog that can in all likelihood be treated!'

Not rooted to the spot as in *informed consent*; as in, 'But he hasn't even discussed the diagnosis and prognosis with them!'

Not rooted to the spot as in *uppity student*; as in, 'The bastard!', or 'What a moron!'

But rooted to the spot as in ... a piece of furniture, a black hole, a free will-free zone, an unquestioning underling-who's-only-obeying-orders.

I'm not even convinced that I managed to squeak out a 'but couldn't we operate on her?' To which he would have replied, in cold and sarcastic incredulity, 'an old bitch like that?' I put up no resistance, and I put the dog down. I anaesthetised her, I euthanised her. All on my own in my consulting room. Dr Vailleux had gone back to his office.

I should have stood up to him, I should have yelled at him, I should have argued with him, I should have stamped my foot, I should have ...

To all intents and purposes, this was my first consultation and my first diagnosis, for a dog at least.

It took me a while to understand what had happened that day. To understand that he was wrong. At the time, it would never have occurred to me to seriously question his decision: I knew he was competent and intelligent. I put the dog down because he told me to.

Of course there was an alternative.

I'd followed his instructions.

Despite the awful leaden feeling in the pit of my stomach, the nausea that I couldn't account for.

I was crushed.

She was dead.

Clémence

'They're so brave, the soldiers.'

She strokes my cheek, takes her hand away and looks at me tenderly, then gives a little skip of happiness and twirls around. She laughs.

I watch her, astonished.

Squatting down beside her dog, I watch her as she skips and twirls.

A woman gives a little embarrassed laugh. A man smiles at her.

Her eyes sparkle.

'Why are you here?'

I crouch on the lawn, in the garden, beneath the plum tree that's losing the last of its blossom, beside her dog that has so much difficulty in standing.

'I'm looking after Follet, Clémence, I'm here to take care of Follet. I'm the vet. The vet. You know?'

She gives a little trill of laughter, mischievous, elegant, the childish laugh that I knew already from the time when I looked after the horde of hamsters that her husband used to keep. She thought keeping hamsters was a bizarre, hare-brained fad for an old gentleman. An old gentleman who was a little lost, a little eccentric. She used to look at him in that same tender, indulgent way, the way you'd look at a child, the way she looked at that soldier long ago. The way she looked at me. A minute ago, or 90 years in the past.

The hamsters are gone now. What happened to them?

What happened to the cats, all of them called Minette (the females) or Minou (the toms)? Minou the grey tom, Minette the black cat with a white patch, Minou the tabby tom, Minette the white cat with a black patch?

Now the only one left is Follet.

Clémence's husband is dead and buried. And her memory with him, perhaps? Clémence, her smiles, her indulgence and her exquisite manners. She still has her laugh – her laugh and her joie de vivre. Her exquisite manners are not those of an old lady, more those of a young girl.

I run my hand over my chin, wonder if I should have shaved. Do I really look like an unshaven soldier from the trenches of the Great War?

There's a lump in my throat.

'And you, Monsieur, why are you here?'

Masculine psychology

Conversation between two vets

'So, what did you invoice for?'

'Well, nothing. I mean, just the vaginal smear to check for sperm, so as not to do an artificial insemination for no reason.'

'And there weren't any?'

'Well, no.'

'And you saw her yesterday?'

'Yes, for the smear, she was just coming into the oestrus phase. Hence the AI today if it didn't work.'

'Yeah, OK, so just the smear on top since it follows on from yesterday, but still, we spent a while there all the same.'

'Well yeah, but I can hardly bill for that!'

'The computer doesn't have a heading for "masturbation".'

'Well no, you moron.'

'Yeah, well I mean, we must have spent, what, half an hour there, the two of us?'

'Well, yeah.'

'For nothing.'

'Well ... I suppose we didn't get anything.'

'We barely managed to produce a hard-on.'

'Yeah, it was annoying.'

'Yeah.'

'Especially as she was up for it.'

'That was obvious. But it's no reason not to invoice.'

'Well, I felt like a complete wally. So I didn't see how I could charge them for that.'

'Well, I dunno, we spent ten minutes explaining to them how to create the best conditions to encourage him to cover her naturally. You could have charged something on that basis.'

'Oh. Yeah, that's not silly.'

'But still, not invoicing is plain daft. Makes it look like we're no good at masturbation, doesn't it?'

'Do you think she'll see it like that?'

'Nah, I shouldn't think so, she's not twisted like us, and anyway she trusts us.'

'For masturbation?'

'Oh stop being such a pillock.'

'Yeah but all the same, the owner of the male said that if he wasn't going to cover her, what was the point of him keeping his balls? Snip, snip.'

'Oh no, it's all my fault!'

'Now you're the one who's being a pillock.'

'Yeah, yeah ...'

Against her will

The silence is suffocating. There are three of us in the half-darkness of the X-ray room.

There's the man. I don't know how he fits into the family exactly. He's leaning against the wall, his hands clasped behind his back, looking up at the ceiling mostly. Now and again he shakes his head, as if in denial, but he opted out of the discussion about half an hour ago.

'It's up to Francette. It's her dog.'

Then there's Madame Rodriguez. Francette. She's in her seventies, with severe glasses, the skin around them etched with hard lines. A tiny, bird-like woman, lips tightly pursed. There's a violence in that mouth, those lines. Could it be anger? Possibly.

And then there's me. Tall, hollow-cheeked, unshaven, in my white coat and dubious footwear. Lost in the middle of the room, I talk to the dog rather than Madame Rodriguez. I find it difficult to look at people when I know we don't agree.

And of course there's Duchesse. She's the reason we're here, a sort of miniature pinscher. Orange-coloured, almost brown under the yellow ceiling light. She's lying on her right side. Her breathing is fast, too fast and too shallow. She's dying.

The room is in shadow. A dimmer lamp on its lowest setting, a negatoscope light box, its glow blotted out by an X-ray. I've just put down the ultrasound probe, the diagnosis is easy. Or at least it is today; a couple of days ago I missed it completely. Duchesse was getting better with the treatment I'd prescribed, she'd started eating again. Then this morning, around six o'clock, she started to whine, and her condition began to deteriorate. Now it's only just ten o'clock, and she's dying. I know why, I know what has to be done. But standing between Duchesse and me is Madame Rodriguez.

I've just given my diagnosis. And my prognosis, broadly. It's very serious, but she also has a serious chance of pulling through. She's no youngster, but at the same time she's only ten. For a pinscher that's not old. But if she's going to live I need to operate, now.

And Madame Rodriguez has just asked me to put her down.

The man is leaning against the wall, looking up at the ceiling. He shakes his head. He picks up his mobile and leaves the room.

I'm stunned. I'm not thinking, I can't any more. I give in. I leave her there, alone with Duchesse. I've turned up the lamp, but the room's still gloomy. I pass one of the nurses, she clocks my expression and says nothing. My mouth must be tightly pursed too. I fetch the euthanasia drugs from the little locked cabinet. My colleague glances at me in alarm.

'You're going to put her down?'

'She doesn't want me to treat her. "Too expensive." I've told her there's an organisation that can help with the cost, and we can spread the payment over six months. She won't have it.'

'Oh.'

At this point I notice the man outside in the car park. He's pacing up and down, waving his left arm about while his right hand clamps his mobile to his ear.

Letting out a sigh, I take a green line from the drawer, and I go back to Duchesse.

'Right. I'm not going to charge you, but I want to do a blood test to see if her kidneys are still working.'

She says nothing. I talk softly to Duchesse, as much to break the silence as to reassure her, even though she's deaf. You treat a dog differently when you speak to it as you work. She doesn't feel the needle, I go off with my millilitre of blood. Three minutes of drumming my fingers on the top of the analyser. Three minutes of clenching my teeth, realising I'm clenching my teeth, unclenching them, reclenching them.

Creatinine level below 0.50 mg/dL.

Absolutely nothing wrong with her kidneys. A bonus point for her prognosis. I go back to the X-ray room, uncertain. In the passageway, Monsieur grabs me by the arm.

'Does she really stand a chance, doctor?'

'I've told you, and I stand by what I said: her chances

are at least one in three. Maybe higher. I can't say any better than that. Her kidneys are good, the procedure to follow is clear. But it has to be done quickly.'

'One in three, hmm? Well. She's got money you know. There's no shortage of that.'

*

I go back into the X-ray room. There's still the sound of Duchesse's breathing, so shallow and rapid. She should be on a drip by now. The man is on my heels, mobile in hand.

'Francette, I've had your daughter on the phone, she says Duchesse must have the operation. She says your husband can pay for it.'

'Oh yes, Jean-Paul can pay all right, that's easy enough. But she's in pain, and she's going to die.'

Her voice is harsh, cold.

I intervene, squatting beside the table to apply a tourniquet, twisting my body to be in line with Duchesse's paw.

'Right. I'm inserting the catheter. She'll need it whatever we decide. If we do nothing she'll die. If I operate I'm not certain I can save her, but she stands a chance. One in three, maybe more. She's not suffering from kidney failure.'

'But she's ten! She's old!'

'Madame Rodriguez, a pinscher can live to fifteen, sixteen, even older. She's not old. In human years she'd be in her sixties. Seventy at most. Doctors in hospitals don't let their patients die because they're seventy.'

'They can't save them all either!'

'No, they can't save them all.'

She can only be about seventy, this woman. Perhaps a little younger.

'You said it was very serious!'

'And I stand by what I said. But we can operate, she could recover without any ill effects, and she could live for another five years. If doctors gave up on treating people with serious illnesses when they still had a third of their lives ahead of them, they wouldn't have much of a work-load left.'

Be convincing, speak calmly, smile but not too much, don't patronise. Her life depends on you striking the right note. Be persuasive, not confrontational.

'I have a suggestion to make. I operate, straight away. There are risks, because she's very ill, but she won't get better with drugs and we've run out of time. I can give her an anaesthetic: I've got all the right equipment, the same as hospitals use, and the anaesthetic gases. There's nothing about the anaesthetic that causes me particular concern. I open her up to see what's going on inside. If it looks bad we stop, I give her the euthanasia drugs while she's asleep, she won't feel a thing, she won't be in pain. For her it will be the same as if I'd put her down without operating, and it won't cost you very much. But if it looks like it could work, I carry on with the operation. Not for the sake of it, but to give her a chance. OK?'

Her mouth is pursed, her fingers clenched on her handbag.

The 'chauffeur', the man who didn't want to get involved, gets back in the driving seat:

'Francette, Pauline's on the phone again. Your daughter. She says the op should go ahead. We should give her a chance. A one-in-three chance is good.'

'Pauline, Pauline, yes, yes, it's all very well for her to say, but the dog's in pain and she's going to die, so she has to be put down. That's the way it is, and I'll get another one.'

The voice on the phone is thin and reedy. I can hear it, we can all hear it, in the silence that is barely disturbed by Duchesse's breathing. The man holds the mobile up, a metre from me, a metre from Madame Rodriguez. The voice comes from a long way off.

'MOTHER! Let the vet do the operation! It's Duchesse! FOR CHRIST'S SAKE!'

Silence. Duchesse's breathing. Without looking at either of them, I pick her up and carry her to the operating theatre. On the way I turn round:

'I'm going to operate straight away. In half an hour or less I'll know how bad it is. Wait in the waiting room for half an hour, OK?'

*

It's half an hour later. The peritonitis was acute, the uterus had ruptured only this morning, probably around six o'clock, when Madame Rodriguez heard Duchesse whining and she vomited. I've used over two litres of sodium chloride to clean out every nook and cranny of the peritoneum and I've inserted a drain. When I started, her rectal temperature was only 35 degrees. She was in a coma, and the operation took over an hour. Ovariohysterectomy, partial resection of the mesentery, flush, flush, flush. Despite all our precautions, by the end of surgery her rectal temperature had fallen to 32 degrees.

She took twelve hours to come round from the anaesthetic. For 48 hours she was in a complete daze, with neurological problems that made me fear the worst. Then she managed to stand up. Then she started to eat.

Five days later she went home.

Duchesse is well. She could equally well have died.

In this case the end doesn't justify the means. Not at all.

Except ...

Freezer

Early days

I'm three. Four, maybe. I've just had a litter of pups, but they've gone. Where are they?

No idea.

For the last three days I've been roaming around a hamlet in south-west France, stealing rubbish from dustbins. People look at me, sometimes they talk to me. I sleep in a lean-to that belongs to one of them. It's a bit cold, but life's good, isn't it?

Today, one of the humans who lives here came up to me again, talking to me nicely and offering me some little dog biscuits. I don't understand much of what he says, but he looks tired, he drags his feet and he's bent over, which makes me feel safe. I can see he likes it when I go up to him quietly, head down, tail wagging.

'So my beauty, no tattoo, eh? We'll ask the vet if you've got a chip.'

A car. A long way. Or maybe not? I dunno, no one knows, no one will ever know. It doesn't worry me in any case, I'm used to it. Abandoned? So what?

I like this house: it's warm, and there are lots of people and interesting smells. And they like it when I wag my tail and put my head down. The food's second to none. The tall man strokes me as he moves me around, so OK, I show him my legs and my ears. He runs a strange machine over me. Three times. Then he shakes his head:

'No, no microchip. No tattoo either. She's just had a litter, she's three or four years old, well cared for. It's strange.'

He squats down beside me.

'The problem, Monsieur, is ... eh, pretty girl? You've got an ugly mug, poor thing. She's an Amstaff, an American Staffordshire terrier, a pit bull type. I'm afraid she fits all the criteria for a "dangerous dog". Plus she's got no identification, she hasn't been spayed, in fact she hasn't got much going for her. I'll have to call the mayor.'

I've spotted a young woman on the other side of the room and I reckon she'll make a proper fuss of me. It's odd, they're all very kind, but they all look a bit bothered. No worries, I'll just lay it on a bit and they'll all adore me.

There you are, the tall one in the white coat is on the phone, talking about me:

'Grey and white, around 40 centimetres tall at the shoulder, a nice plump, well-fed Amstaff. Yes, she's been roaming around a hamlet in your area for three days. Yes, it's a female, just had pups, no identification.'

No identification, but still a bit of a looker, with my close-cropped coat, my ash-blonde colouring, my brown eyes, my great lolloping tongue and the way I'm always up for a bit of fun and games. A three-year-old kid, really. Pretty, with an ugly mug. I must remember that, it'll look good on my pedigree.

'We'll keep her for a few days for you before she's sent to the pound, in case her owner turns up. But I doubt if he will: she's illegal and he knows it. Anyway, I'll keep you in the picture. She seems pretty good-natured, so there shouldn't be any problem.

'Yes, legally you can ask for her to be put down at any time.

'Yes, I realise you don't kill a dog just like that, but I'm informing you, and you are responsible for her after all ...'

His voice trails off, the tall one in the white coat. They all look at me from the top of legs that go on for ever, hands on hips or arms folded.

'Well now, what are we going to do with you?'

Wag that tail.

Paradise

No, seriously, it's true: every morning they feed me, then someone takes me out for a walk. Little by little they're starting to trust me, and when there's no one around they let me off the lead in a big field. It's more practical, in any case. Then they tie my lead to a cupboard near the office, with a blanket – if there's no blanket I bark like crazy, I'm not going to be messed around, am I? – and I spend the day snoring, snuffling, eating, drinking, having a fuss made of me.

The good life.

You have to work at it, though: sometimes these humans can be pretty dim. Sometimes they leave me alone for a couple of minutes or more, or they don't make a fuss of me, or they ignore me even! Whenever they do that I kick up an almighty fuss, whining and whimpering – not just ordinary barking, more a kind of squeaky, rasping noise that's brilliant at getting a reaction, and fast. Then they shout all sorts of things at me, give me lots of attention and stop ignoring me. Bliss.

'Oh for pity's sake will you just shut UP!'

'Someone put a muzzle on it! Goddammit!'

'Doesn't she *ever* stop?'

'You're a lovely girl, a pretty girl, but you've got an ugly mug and you're a pain in the bum, aren't you?'

'Behave, or we'll put you in the freezer!'

When they all come running, red in the face, shouting at me and shaking me a bit, I go into my routine: wag the tail, look blissfully happy. It comes naturally.

'Oh god, she's so dumb, and she's so lovable, but whatever are we going to do with her?'

The young woman goes away on a fortnight's holiday. Just before she leaves she puts a note on my cage:

'She's so adorable, look after her, find her a good home, see you in a fortnight.'

Sweet of her, don't you think? The guys in white coats loved it when they found it on the Monday morning. They looked even more nonplussed than usual. It set them talking. Which meant they were five minutes late with my breakfast. Not good.

Not good at all.

So I went into my whining act.

'Aaaargggh, no, stop it! If you don't behave we'll put you in the freezer!'

But I got my breakfast and my walk, and they made a fuss of me.

Freezer

'I called the Society for the Protection of Animals. They don't want her. They say they won't be allowed to rehome her because of her "dangerous dog" status, so either she'll moulder away in their kennels or they'll have to put her down. Yeah, the mayor agrees that we can keep her for the moment, we'll try to find her a good home.'

They've even given me a name. I like it, it's punchy, it sounds good, and I bet there aren't any other dogs called 'Freezer'.

I watch as a lot of people come and go. Some of them come to see me, but most of them just happen to be here with their own dogs – I'm not allowed to play with them – and start talking about me with the guys in white coats.

'She's a sweet dog, has she been abandoned?'

Did he say sweet? Wag tail, head down, make a fuss of him. They love it, fuss guaranteed.

'Yup.'

'What breed is she?'

'What would you say?'

'I dunno, um, a boxer?'

'No, no way, boxers are completely different. She's more like an Amstaff, a pit bull.'

'A pit bull? But she's not dangerous!'

No, course not. Adorable, clingy, whiny, tiresome, boisterous, but not dangerous. And pretty!

The guy in the white coat says that at least I'll have shown lots of people that pit bulls aren't necessarily dangerous dogs. It shatters the myth, he says. It lays a few ghosts, and it's an opportunity to show people the true consequences of paying lip-service to presidential declarations, and to rub their noses in it.

I'm not a ghost, like he says. I'm not bothered, I'm getting good food, I'm getting a fuss made of me, and when there's no one around I can wander round the clinic.

Lots of people have come in and said they'd find me a home. Old people, young people, English people, French people, people in comfortable clothes and people in not so comfortable clothes, people who smell of cows and people who smell of perfume. Will they find me a home?

Whatever. None of them ever come back anyway.

The guys in white coats talk a lot, and make lots of phone calls. They still look nonplussed when they see me, so I wag my tail. You can't beat it. Well, sometimes when I go a bit over the top with the whining they don't look nonplussed at all, but well, I'm bored stiff, what do they expect!'

'Freezer, shut UP!'

Seriously.

Three weeks it's gone on now. It's evening, and the taller guy in the white coat is squatting beside me, a cigarette between his lips, watching me as I roll on the grass. He looks sad.

'The condemned man's last cigarette, hmm?'

There were loads of phone calls this afternoon. I even saw the mayor, though the mayor didn't really want to see me.

A really nice lady asked the vets if they were going to 'euthanise' me:

'Surely you're not going to?'

'Are you offering to have her?'

Silence ...

'But doesn't it seem strange to you to kill a healthy, good-natured three-year-old dog that's been part of your daily life for the past three weeks?'

The guy in the white coat looked at her. Then he put on a weird voice:

'You vets do such a *won*derful job.'

I'm not bothered, I'm rolling in the grass. It's cold. Life's good.

'I'm sorry, pretty girl, you've got an ugly mug.'

Wag that tail.

I get a whole shed-load of cuddles and strokes on their funny table. I didn't much like that plastic needle thing they put in my paw, and they don't say anything, or not much, but they make a big fuss of me. And they mean it.

I'm pretty, I'm lovable, I'm clingy and I'm a bit of a pain in the bum.

They're all here: wag that tail.

The guy in the white coat is holding a syringe, and his expression is blank. They stroke me as he gives me the injection.

I'm pretty, I'm lovable, I'm clingy and I'm a bit of a pain in the bum. I'm called ...

Freezer.

Birth

It's darkest night. The moon is completely hidden behind the clouds, but my headlights sweep across the surreal sight of this little forest road in the middle of a hailstorm. A carpet of leaves covers the road, lime green and silver with the tarred surface peeping through here and there, streaming with water, black and dazzling in the glare of the halogen beams.

Among the bushes that rush past at such hectic speed I make out thickets of young branches and leaves, ferns and brambles, impenetrable refuges for deer no doubt terrified by the storm.

The orange display on the dashboard tells me it's one o'clock in the morning.

The air is cool, yet it's mild outside, with not a breath of wind. The damp smell of woodland lingers on the air. I feel as though I'm floating on a soft cloud of sensations washed clean by the storm. Ten minutes ago I was oblivious to the weather. I was fast asleep, cocooned in the duvet, far away from the world and its storms.

A man comes towards me. A retired farmer who fifteen

years ago had his moment of glory with a herd that regularly swept the board at agricultural shows. Even in Paris.

Now I'd be hard pushed to put an age to him. If I didn't know he was retired, I'd say he was barely 60. He sighs, recites a little monologue, tells me he's made a mistake, that he should never have let this pregnancy go to full term when the heifer is barely two years old. An accident.

'She was there beside me, chewing the cud, looking at me. Her waters had broken an hour earlier, and then nothing, she wasn't straining. I put my hand inside her and the calf was dead, all stiff.'

Somewhere inside me an impossible hope stirs, a voice whispers that the calf will come out by itself, even if the heifer is young, even if she's too fat, even if out of the three calvings this retired farmer has had – and there have only been three – we've had to intervene three times. The fourth will be different ...

The cow is lying in a large calving box, on a deep bed of fresh straw. Beyond the barrier that separates the box from the rest of the cowshed, an enormous blonde cow is twisting round to get a better view. Beside her is the calf, too large and too heavy, that I helped her deliver barely two weeks ago. I'd suggested then that we should induce the heifer that night. He'd decided to wait.

The adrenalin hasn't kicked in yet, and I feel a bit anaesthetised. I pull off my jumper, put on my waterproof apron and examination gloves, and pass the caesarean box with its resuscitation equipment under the barrier. I also grab the calving aid and some ropes.

'Can you hold the cow?'

'She won't budge ...'

I climb over the barrier and slip my right hand into the birth canal of the cow, which is still lying down and watches me curiously. My left hand is leaning on her leg, my knees are sunk in the straw. The calf is a big one, the birth canal isn't fully dilated, nor is the cervix. I pinch the skin between the calf's hooves. No reaction. Yes, it probably is dead.

'Right, let's tie her up and get her on her feet, then we can see if it'll pass.'

I feel as though it's an effort to raise my voice, yet the air is so pure that according to all the clichés it should slice clean through the ether like the crack of whip, the shaft of an arrow, a chord of crystalline notes or whatever else you care to mention. I feel really groggy, insubstantial: I'm going to have to concentrate.

When she sees the farmer's rope, the young cow grasps right away that things are getting serious. She gets up by herself, and walks round the box a couple of times for form's sake, before giving in and letting us get on with what we have to do.

This time I try to muster a little more energy. Surely I can manage to shake off my torpor now? Both arms deep inside her, I check how much further the birth canal and vulva can dilate. For the moment, the calf won't get through. Despite the stimulation, the cow doesn't strain: another lazy one that will have to have it all done for her. The calf, meanwhile, seems well and truly dead. Oh well, we'll see ...

I get down to work, moving my arms back and forth to force the cow to strain, to push the calf upwards. Its hooves aren't even pointing forwards, the cervix is still far too evident, the birth canal too narrow, and I'm not even sure that the cow's pelvis is wide enough to allow the calf to pass through. A C-section for a dead calf, though ... I'll give it my best shot, anyway, I just want to get back to bed as soon as I can. Very slowly, as I push and pull my arms back and forth, back and forth, the cow starts to respond, contracting her abdomen and pushing a little, again just for form's sake. Not enough. Gradually the scent of the forest is submerged by the sickly smell of amniotic fluid, and I feel as though I'm enclosed in a bubble of straw, its circumference described by the golden light of the little light bulb hanging on the wall. It's very dark. Beyond the windbreak netting I sense the presence of the Pyrenees, but it's all unreal. There's just the cow and me. Apart from her breathing, the pauses when she pushes, and my encouragements to her, nothing disturbs the silence of the night. I've almost forgotten about the farmer. We're in for the long haul. Seriously long.

At last, after I've been working away for ten minutes or so, I emerge from my comfortable cocoon. I'm awake at last. My forehead is beaded with sweat. The cow has also shrugged off her bovine torpor. We both surface from our trance-like state in synchrony, moving slowly in a strange dance, to the syncopated beat of our joint exertions. Waves of amniotic-laden air submerge and engulf me. There's the cow, the calf, and me.

'So?'

One word from the farmer and the spell is broken. I pause in my efforts. Immediately, the heifer stops pushing.

'Let's attach the ropes and give it a try. I don't think it'll work, though.'

I position the two nooses: the hooves are pointing towards the vulva at last, but the head hasn't even passed through the pelvis. As the calving aid starts to pull, the cow lies down, but despite our efforts not even the head is engaged. Abruptly I call a halt.

'It won't come out. We'll have to open her up.'

The expression on the farmer's face speaks volumes. His lips move:

'Bugger.'

I couldn't agree more. It's nearly twenty past one. Only twenty past one?

'I'll call my neighbour and ask him to bring the clippers over.'

'Very good. I'll get everything ready.'

Open the caesarean box, check the suture materials, get out the antibiotics and an injection of tocolytics, an anti-contraction medication. Now what?

Wait.

Five long minutes after I've laid everything out, the neighbour arrives. It's all I can do not to sink back into my slumbers.

Shave, clean, disinfect, now things are getting serious. Despite the odd kick from the cow, which doesn't appreciate the injections of local anaesthetic, the atmosphere remains serenely calm: even the neighbour has now slipped inside our cotton-wool cocoon. I don't pay much attention to his small talk about the hailstorm, any more than I do to the protestations of the heifer, which after our combined efforts of earlier seems to view the ordeal I'm now subjecting her to as a betrayal. OK, now I'm descending into anthropomorphism. It really is time to go back to bed.

I make an incision in the hide. This time the heifer doesn't move.

A few strokes of the scalpel, light as caresses, and the muscles of her flank part. She gazes at me inscrutably. The way the muscular fibres unzip in a stream of blood, without the slightest effort on my part, is almost surreal.

Now there's just the last membrane, the fine milky wall behind which I can feel the slow contraction and warmth of the intestines. The peritoneum. One final stroke, light as a feather, and I put down the scalpel. I disinfect my gloves one last time, then sink my left arm into the heifer's belly. Still she doesn't move. I skirt round the rumen and slip my hand under the uterus. I can feel the calf's hocks through the uterus, which feels reassuringly solid: it won't tear.

I draw my arm out, before plunging it back in, this time with an ordinary paper knife in my hand. I locate the hocks, and prick the uterus with the point of the paper knife. Working blind, I feel the tissues in the depths of the cow's abdomen slide apart almost imperceptibly. The opening is large enough. I draw my hand out and put down the paper knife. The two retired farmers stand ready to attach the ropes to the calf's hind legs. I don't need to say a word: between us we have a certain amount of experience of these births.

My hand slips into the mother's belly to find my incision again. I take hold of the calf's hock, and I pinch it – just in case. I have to hide a grin. There was a reaction. It's alive, but I don't say anything. I don't want to build up any false hopes only to dash them again. In any case, in a minute it will be out. I follow the cannon bone with my hand to reach the hoof of the right hind leg, which I draw towards the opening in the uterus and then towards myself, towards the outside world. The uterus follows in a harmonious rocking motion, the hoof punctures the amniotic sac, the older of the two farmers has already got his rope in place and is holding the hoof outside.

When he exclaims, 'But it's moving!', I don't respond. I'm already drawing out the second hoof, to be held in place by an expertly placed rope, not touching the edge of the wound. Perfect.

'Yes, it's alive! Let's get it out, come on, upwards and backwards!'

They make quite a sight, those two old boys, as they toil away in a frenzy, straining with all their might in this awkward movement that's designed to allow the calf to unfold itself and us to get it out without exerting any unnecessary pressure on the uterus. To help them in their efforts, I enlarge the incision in the skin and muscles slightly: I'd made it a little too tight, as always. The two veterans pant away, the calf emerges slowly, very slowly. There's a wave of relief as its pelvis passes through the wound: the rest is just a formality. I break its fall by cradling it in my arms, then quickly lower it to the ground. It's huge, but it's alive.

I rip off my gloves, still lost in a strange trance-like state. I check the umbilical cord, grab the cardio-respiratory analeptics – the stimulants: it's stopped breathing.

'Suspend it, quickly!'

The first farmer clambers over the barrier to slide the rope through the pulley that's already in position, while the other one ties it around the nooses that are still attached to the calf's hind legs. I help them to suspend it upside down, clear the airways quickly, then give it an intravenous injection into the jugular of a drug strong enough to bring it back from the dead.

Before it has time to take its first breath I start on cardiac massage, while on my instructions the neighbour sloshes a bucket of ice-cold water in the newborn's face. Welcome to the world!

It takes its first breath, its heart hammering away in response to the stress that's saved its life. It struggles in panicky silence as I carry on extracting the mucus, pushing my fingers down into its trachea. It can come back down to earth now. Already I'm turning away from the calf to take care of its mother, who's gazing at us as though we were extraterrestrials from some schlocky B-movie, spattered with blood, with straw in our hair and spouting top-quality dialogue:

'Oh my god! Oh my god! If it isn't alive! Jesus, Mary and Joseph! Good lord above!'

If he'd been younger, obviously, it would have been something more along the lines of 'shit shit shit'. Plus ça change.

Meanwhile I'm working out what I still have to do. The uterine incision is pretty clean and the uterus isn't torn, so that should be OK. I wedge the uterus on the side of the wound and start suturing.

First a continuous suture to close it up. I check it's tight enough and watertight. I think I must have woken up at the same time as the calf. When I resuscitated it we must have shared the same adrenalin rush. Now I share banter and sympathy with the farmer, who will have to ensure the survival of this enormous calf that looks every bit as lively as its mother ...

A good twenty minutes later the second continuous suture is done, to ensure the uterus is properly sealed and bury the suture. This uterus wasn't so easy to stitch up in the end.

I like the way the uterus looks after all those stitches, almost as if nothing had happened at all. Finally, I put the uterus back in place. Already it's shrunk massively in size.

Suture of the peritoneum and first muscular layer. There's a lot of meat on this animal.

Suture of the next two muscular layers, no problem. In comparison with the suture of the uterus, these are a mere formality.

Finally, I sew up the hide and close the wound.

It's three o'clock in the morning. Now that I'm wide awake, I can go back to bed.

Or else I'll have a coffee with the two old boys, and a match replay. The calf is alive in the end, but he's looking just about as alert as I probably did when I arrived earlier.

The night is still silent, still starless.

Go on then, time for that coffee.

Failure

Failure is an old friend of mine, always looking over my shoulder, always ready to catch me out with some unforeseen twist, some new and grim practical joke. Failure haunts me whenever I carry out an examination, whenever I make a diagnosis, whenever I give a treatment, whenever I do a dissection or make a ligature. Failure clocks all my mental blanks and stupid mistakes, feeds my anxieties and multiplies my doubts.

Failure propels me forwards, too, driving me on to research subjects more deeply through the pages of medical books and the arcane hinterland of the internet. Failure sends me back to the drawing board, forces me to reconsider, quite simply teaches me to learn.

Failure is a constant companion in my daily routine. I try to keep the upper hand, by checking and observing, phoning and warning. Keep an eye on your pet, Monsieur: if you see this, or you don't see that, call me, make an appointment, bring him back to see me. And if all's well, give me a call to let me know. Nowadays the charge for many of the operations I carry out includes a follow-up appointment, well before the stitches come out. For cases of ear infections and corneal ulcers there are always several follow-up appointments, at a reduced rate or even virtually free if there are a lot of them.

Whenever anything takes an unexpected turn, I go back to my diagnosis, try to find the flaw in the treatment: was it the wrong treatment, or was it the right treatment wrongly applied? Has the owner administered the ear drops so that they penetrate into the inner ear, or has she deposited them in the outer ear, for fear of hurting her pet? A demonstration, a discussion around the subject, a check on the amount of liquid left – all can be useful avenues to explore. Further tests, ruled out initially, can be done. Bacterial and antibiotic susceptibility tests, for instance. Or X-rays, who knows?

Often, failure takes no account of the knock-on effects it can unleash; at its worst, it can set back healing, delay a cure.

And sometimes failure can kill.

Occasionally failure is my fault, the result of a mistake on my part. Insufficient knowledge or the wrong interpretation of a sign or symptom can lead to a false or incomplete diagnosis. Sometimes you can't see the wood for the trees. Or you put your finger on the effect and then confuse it with the cause. Failure rarely comes as a surprise: the more experienced I become, the more easily I can spot the underhand tricks and betrayals that it keeps in store. The better I can prepare for it, the better I can prepare the owner to recognise it, and together we can turn it into another step on the way to diagnosis and treatment. If I continue to foster my doubts, and my anxieties, this sort of failure will wither on the vine and die.

Sometimes the failure is on the owner's part. There are owners who refuse to accept a diagnosis of an illness, or the treatment for it, because of their own convictions, their own fears. In these cases I have to explain my reasoning, dissect it, justify it, occasionally resort to being manipulative. Make them understand the consequences of their decisions, of their awkwardness. Get things back on track, if I can. The longer this type of failure goes on, the more it becomes my own failure. I appropriate it to myself jealously, snatch it away from the irresponsible owner, accuse and condemn myself. I am judge and jury, I act as my own prosecution and my own defence. I should have seen it coming, I should have guessed, I forgot to make it clear. They couldn't have known, they must have misunderstood, it's all my fault. This type of failure wears you down, dragging you into lengthy explanations, prevarications, precautions, justifications. I need to sustain the support and commitment of the owner and their family, nurture and maintain their motivation, be aware that you can say something one way to one person, but you need to say it quite differently to another – with all the risks that go with this of losing the plot, of losing myself, or of losing the person I'm trying to protect. Too much explanation is self-defeating, and after the lengthiest ones I always finish up by saying: 'I've deluged you with information, I know, and it's not all straightforward. If you'd like me to explain more, or if you have any questions, don't hesitate to call me.'

And then there are the times when failure can be laid neither at my door nor at the owner's.

This is when it's the failure of a system. Money, or the lack of it, invariably places restrictions on the possible treatments we can explore: therein lies one of the fundamental differences between veterinary medicine and human medicine as practised in France and other European countries. How much is a diagnosis worth, whether for a simple infection or for a serious illness? Or if it condemns an animal to certain death, or to a lingering and painful demise? Or if it doesn't even lead to treatment, as there's no point? How much is a life worth? This type of failure is by its very nature unfair. It may be possible to rationalise it, to justify it, but – unless you take refuge in cynicism or harden your heart – it's still monstrous. So you have to accept it and find ways round it. Whenever I can, I offer staged payments, a discount, or some other solution. Sometimes I even offer treatment for free. But an animal is still an animal. However abhorrent we may find this sort of failure, we should never forget that.

Failure can also be laid at the door of society, and of its stupidity, for which we all bear a responsibility. Like putting down a dog that's done nothing to deserve it, for instance. I try to negotiate a way round such cases, to limit the damage – but at what cost? How many other responsibilities does this endanger? In a modest way I try to make a difference, and it makes me shiver when I read about

– when I have to live through – failures of this sort, which never 'just' affect the animals concerned.

Finally, failure can simply signal our impotence in the face of illness, or of death. Natural and ineluctable, clearly this failure is the easiest to accept – although this doesn't necessarily make it any easier to bear.

No dialysis or kidney transplant for an animal suffering from kidney failure, just pain and loneliness.

No more analgesics for terminal arthritis, pain or paralysis. No more playing, no more pirouettes.

No more antibiotics against bacteria, now victorious, resistant, immortal.

With the passage of time, these failures become harder to bear, more violent to endure. Because I used to be a locum, or an assistant, safely behind the scenes, veiled in obscurity. There were pillars behind which I could hide, or prevaricate; there were other people on whom I could lean. Animals were cases, always new, and their owners were strangers.

But time passes.

Now I'm not on my own, but other people count on me, lean on me. And I'm not ready for it, not yet! Gone are the days when I could listen to the words of a wise mentor, put blind faith in him or her. Now I view the opinions of my peers with a creeping doubt, the doubt that's essential to every diagnosis, every decision. I've lost that blithe confidence and trust, and there can be no doubt whatever that my patients are better off for it.

A doctor who was coming up to retirement used to tell

me that his patients were ageing with him, and that now they would be dying.

So what about three-year-old Corneille, who's dying tonight?

I witnessed his first steps, I bandaged his broken paw when he fell down the stairs. I entrusted him to the care of my colleagues for his fracture, his eye problems, his skin infections. I was with him when his owners hatched up crazy schemes to make him a father, dreams that were never to be realised. I was there when his intended paramour arrived on the scene, forever to remain his platonic friend. I reassured his mistress, encouraged his master. Corneille always had something wrong, and over time we made a good team. Now his bumps and bruises are gone, his wretched soft palate is gone, the pink tip of his tongue that always vanished when I tried to get hold of it, all are gone. Because a bacterial infection decided to become resistant. A 'banal' skin infection.

So as not to cry, I focused on listening to his heartbeat as it weakened tonight, to his heartbeat as it fibrillated, then stopped.

A failure, but one that we accept, that we can justify, that no one can reproach themselves for. But no less devastating for all that, no less painful.

Silky

He's a farmer, with a hundred or so head of cattle. In his fifties, with four children and stepchildren. The oldest boy is set to take over the farm, and is already finding his place there. The farmer reflects on things, thinks ahead, develops his herd, keeps abreast of the latest methods.

But he's not optimistic, all the same.

He can't see a future for his farm. 'Children? They're mollycoddled, over-indulged. How can you expect them to work when they already have everything? At their age I had nothing.'

He leans on his stick, cap on head, watching the drip flow.

'Oh, my wife wants you to go and see that wretched animal. If only it would give up the ghost! It's not like a blasted cat. They don't need any looking after, do they!'

I follow his gaze to the seat of his tractor, where his favourite kitten used to sit, the one that he used to carry around under his cap. That got run over. That he misses.

'What a charrracter! Extrrraordinarrry!'

Not even the legendary local singer Claude Nougaro,

whose accent you could cut with a knife, rolled his 'r's with such extravagance.

'He'll soon be costing us more than a calf does, that stupid animal.'

'The guinea pig?'

'What a waste of space!'

*

It doesn't cost you anything, as you know full well. It was you who brought it to me. When you brought it to the surgery with your youngest son and he said, 'It's going to die, it'll have to be put down', it was you I heard in the car just beforehand, putting him up to it.

When I suggested that I should operate instead, for the same price as putting it down, and if it didn't work to put it down anyway, you allowed yourself to be persuaded with good grace. And when your son said again, 'It's going to die, it'll have to be put down', you even swatted him lightly on the head and said, 'Come on, son, leave the vet in peace to get on with his work.'

I gave Quenotte an anaesthetic, lanced and cleaned its abscess, filed its teeth. I even did an X-ray, to be sure. It was bad, it would get worse again. Then I took it home for the weekend. To hand-feed it, get it back on its feet.

It was Madame who came to fetch it. I told her that its life was saved, for the moment.

'You'll have to carry on hand-feeding it, as you have been already. It's not in pain now, so it should be easier. You'll need to give it these antibiotics, and this for the pain.

And obviously it's not over. Not by a long way. The roots of the teeth are at an angle, they'll never grow straight, they'll need regular clipping. Maybe as often as once a fortnight.'

She paid what it would have cost to put it down, as agreed. Then I was a step ahead of her.

'I know your husband will complain because we'll need to see it so often and you'll often have to hand-feed it. And how much will the darn thing cost! So you can tell him that for one thing, my two-year-old daughter has been feeding it for the past two days, and she's called it Silky. And for another thing, I won't charge you for filing its teeth, only for the medication and food.'

*

She never really accepted this gift. And since she couldn't bring herself to accept it, she took it upon herself bring us little cakes, biscuits and other delicious treats. Because she knew that we at least appreciated the cakes and gateaux she would always offer us with our coffee after a calving or a transfusion. It was an arrangement that suited all us vets at the surgery extremely well.

*

So you can see we're not about to let that guinea pig give up the ghost.

Not on your life.

Her hand on my arm

Her call had been a sob and a cry, urgent, instinctive, incoherent. I've never been able to recall what she said, I just remember dropping the drawer of resuscitation meds, abandoning the appointment I was in the middle of, flinging myself in the car, and almost ploughing into the wall of her house, barely a couple of hundred metres from the surgery.

She used to refer to us as her 'cruise'. Every week, virtually, she would come to fetch medication for Boule's heart. Boule was some sort of labrador cross, big and solid, easy-going and imperturbable. His heart was rubbish, his heartbeat a drumbox mix of dub, reggae, waltz and disco. Every time she came to pick up his pills for the following week she'd chat to us about Boule, about the weather, and especially about the cruise that she would never go on.

I think she came every week in order to avoid having to write any 'big' cheques.

I sprinted out of the car, stethoscope in one hand, box of medication and syringes in the other. She pointed towards the laurel hedge. She was in tears. Boule wasn't lying down, he'd fallen down. All I could see was his ample rear end, the tail that I'd only ever seen wagging now lying still.

No pulse, no heartbeat, I gave him heart massage, inserted the tracheal tube as never before.

She was crying. He'd jumped up out of the blue, run outside, fallen down.

Much later I heard that her family, though she never mentioned them, had parked her here, in this little village in the middle of nowhere, when she'd followed them to the south of France from her own village in faraway Alsace. She hadn't followed them a second time. She'd kept her house, Boule, her few friends and her solitude. And her dreams of going on a cruise. To the Caribbean, or the Pacific, Madagascar or Réunion, the Windward Islands or the lagoons of New Caledonia.

Whenever she signed a cheque she'd look at us with a wistful smile; each time it was 'a little bit of her cruise'.

Boule used to hate coming to see us at the surgery.

Now he'd stopped breathing, but only just.

I put the ligature in place, picked up the catheter.

She put her hand on my arm.

'Has he gone?'

He'd gone, but only just.

'Then leave him be, doctor.'

She put her hand on my arm, and I sat down heavily on my backside like an idiot, and it was all I could do stop myself from crying.

*

She never did go on her cruise.

'Oh cruises, they're full of boring old farts who've never had a Boule.'

The last calf

The mobile rings.

It's 8.35 in the morning and I'm on call, but the surgery opens at nine. Probably someone else wanting an appointment. I'm not even going to bother to answer. If it's urgent they'll leave a message. If not, they'll call back.

And there it goes, the beep-beep-beep of a voice message. Most likely just the click of someone ringing off.

'Oh. He says he's out on call, what shall I do?'

She's holding the phone away from her face, I imagine her arm dangling. I hear a second voice behind her. I can see her standing in the doorway to her house, I know who she is already.

'Oh. Well, leave a message?'

Just what I was going to say.

'Yes, hello, it's Madame Colucci, it's about a calving, it's twins and they're both breech, it's urgent.'

I'm already in the car. On the way the mobile rings again, same number. I confirm that I've got the message and I'm on my way. Within ten minutes of her call I'm there.

*

As I park the vehicle and undo my seatbelt in a single move, the heavy door to the cowshed slides open. I'm already rummaging in the boot as Monsieur and Madame Colucci emerge, trudging over with a heavy tread. I'm already kitted out in calving apron and examination gloves, 'birthing box' in hand, as I remove my head from the boot to say hello. I bid them a bright and breezy hello, which proves to be startlingly at odds with the doleful expressions they're wearing.

On the way to the cowshed I learn that the cow is old-but-not-that-old, that she's a good size, and that Monsieur thinks it's twins because there's a head and there are hind feet. He only mentions about ten times that of course he can't be certain of this, in a tone of voice that makes it perfectly clear that in fact he's in no doubt at all.

It's only when I reach the doorway that I remember what I'd forgotten.

A blonde cow is gazing at me, her tail comically raised for a contraction. She's certainly big. And she looks as if she's doing just fine. It's the pair of heifers waiting at the other end of the big building that drag me back to the sad reality of the situation, however. A month ago, Monsieur and Madame Colucci's herd was dispersed and sold. Now there are just three animals left. There's someone else there, someone I don't know, a neighbour I assume. I say hello absent-mindedly. Then they tell me that he's come to collect the cow.

There's a bit of a lump in my throat. It's a long way from the jovial atmosphere I'm used to at calvings where you have an instinct that all will go well, where experience and observation, obstetric manipulation and sheer physical effort come together, where there's no risk of a caesarean, no danger to the cow, and probably none to the calf either.

Madame – sturdily built and an imposing figure in her blue-and-white striped housecoat, her hair gathered in improbable bunches – rather overshadows her husband, a slight figure in his blue overalls. They are breeders of calves reared by their mothers, whose products used to clean up all the prizes at every agricultural show. As reliable and unchanging as the Pyrenees.

It isn't twins. The calf is on its back, feet in the air, and those are indeed the hind legs. It's the position they're in that made Monsieur Colucci and the buyer confuse the calf's knees with its hocks. A classic mistake. The birth passage is wide, the cervix is dilated, there's just a slight torsion that's soon sorted. The calf is alive.

It's the sort of calving I love best, the combined efforts of manual traction and the mother's pushing, working in concert and without the use of a calving jack or aid; the sort of calving from which you emerge with your nostrils filled with the smell of amniotic fluid, your ears deafened by the cow's lowing, your eyes dazzled by the image of the newborn calf shaking its head indignantly as it receives its first bucket of icy water full in the face. The smell of straw and manure, the cool morning air on your bare arms, and washing your hands in icy cold water with Savon de Marseille and a spotlessly clean hand towel.

One of those calvings that you want to share, that are everything I love about this job. One of those perfect calvings, if it weren't for the things that are missing: the typical commotion struck up by other inquisitive members of the herd, the blasé indifference of the seasoned matrons, the deft tongues of the calves as they try to grab my overalls through the bars of their box.

One of those perfect calvings, if it weren't for Madame Colucci's tears, incongruous and startling, coursing down her cheeks at a volume to match her bulk and her bunches. Madame Colucci rubbing her eyes and apologising in the heartbroken voice of a small girl, while her husband looks on with the mournful expression you reserve for the funerals of friends.

If it weren't for the buyer, in his black overalls, looking sheepish and unobtrusive.

And if it weren't for me, the vet, here for what will certainly be the last time, privileged to be a part of, and to witness, this little slice of human history, wondering with a heavy heart when it will be my turn. Me, the vet, wanting more than anything to just sit down in the straw, to pull this calf to me and hold it tight.

As if we've read each other's thoughts, Madame Colucci does it for me.

There's only one of us here who's not musing on the old days.

Who shakes his head, with his great dark doe eyes and his damp, matted coat, struggling already to get to his feet, his instincts kicking in with dazzling, demented speed, gawky and bursting with the will to live.

His mother licks him with a passion.

The last calf.